BALD
LIKE
ME

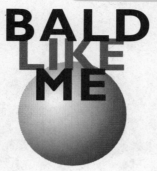

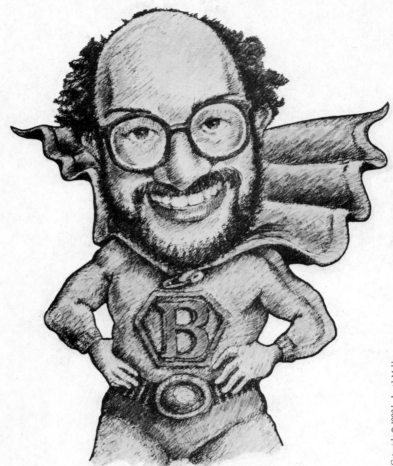

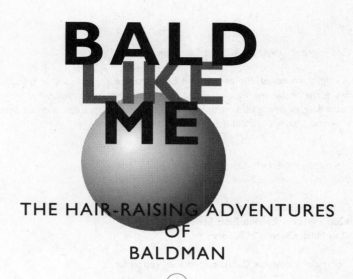

BALD
LIKE
ME

THE HAIR-RAISING ADVENTURES
OF
BALDMAN

RICHARD SANDOMIR

COLLIER BOOKS / MACMILLAN PUBLISHING COMPANY / NEW YORK
COLLIER MACMILLAN CANADA / TORONTO
MAXWELL MACMILLAN INTERNATIONAL
NEW YORK / OXFORD / SINGAPORE / SYDNEY

Collier Books
Macmillan Publishing Company
866 Third Avenue, New York, NY 10022

Collier Macmillan Canada
1200 Eglinton Avenue East, Suite 200
Don Mills, Ontario M3C 3N1

Library of Congress Cataloging-in-Publication Data

Sandomir, Richard.
    Bald like me : the hair-raising adventures of Baldman/by Richard
Sandomir. — 1st Collier Books ed.
        p.   cm.
    ISBN 0-02-036650-7
    1. Baldness—Humor. I. Title
    PN6231.B27S26 1990   90-1780 CIP
    818'.5402–dc20

Macmillan books are available at special discounts for bulk purchases for sales promotions, premiums, fund-raising, or educational use. For details, contact:

    Special Sales Director
    Macmillan Publishing Company
    866 Third Avenue
    New York, NY 10022

10 9 8 7 6 5 6 4 3 2 1

Printed in the United States of America

First Collier Books Edition 1990

CONTENTS

PREFACE

HOW *BALD LIKE ME* CAME TO BE

THIS BOOK HAD its genesis in a column written a few years ago in *New York Newsday*. I was riding to work on the subway when I came upon the overhaired ravings of columnist Denis Hamill, who was lamely describing a meeting of lawyers during an American Bar Association convention. Using his unformed powers of description, Hamill wrote that all the lawyers in attendance were "chrome domes," and any stray guys with hair "had uncles in the carpet business."

This jolted me way beneath the scalp. Sure, I'd heard bald epithets before. Sure, "chrome dome" was commonly used to describe a head bare of hair (though I've yet to see chrome of any sort on a bald head). But this may have been the first time that I felt genuinely insulted by an outsider. I was, until that time, consumed inwardly by my baldness, combing over my loss and looking in every store window I passed to make sure the hair spray kept things under control. But I hadn't focused on the external threat posed by the haired class.

Only now did these insulting descriptions make my scalp burn. What did he know of being bald? What did he know of how his words, so injudiciously chosen, would sting?

Shakespeare, the world's greatest bald playwright, might have opined (had Shylock been bald): "I am a bald man. Hath not a bald man a heart? Hath not a bald man hands, organs, dimensions, senses, affections, passions. If you prick our pate, do we not bleed?"

Reading Hamill, I sweated profusely—and I was riding an air-conditioned subway car. This cruelly cavalier attitude toward the unhaired could not go unavenged. I wrote a letter to Hamill indicating that even the worst toupees are made of different stuff than Kaufman Carpet shag. But he never replied. So I resolved to do more, though I knew my enemy was strong and outhaired me. I knew that when haired bigots rear their ugly manes, they do so without compunction.

And so, the idea for this book took form. I thought of several ways to do it, and rejected pure revenge as overly vindictive. Why should I be as mean-spirited as those who would insult me and my bald brothers? Over the past few years, I've felt that bald and balding men needed to be able to laugh at their haired foes, as well as themselves, and to feel that they have support. We are 30 million strong in this country, an influential voting bloc should Joe Garagiola or Rob Reiner run for president. As I now realize, there is no shame in being bald—nor has there ever been.

Out of my ruminations came *Bald Like Me*, a love letter to my unhaired brethren all over, a way to tell my bald pals, "We're in this together."

On the road to this book's publication, there was a haired conspiracy to reject it, a cabal shunned by the good folks at Macmillan (praise Yul Brynner!). But a conspiracy it was: how else to explain why nineteen other publishers turned it down? One prominent overhaired senior editor of a major publishing house revealed that there were no bald executives with any influence in the entire company, a situation that rendered moot their publishing a baldness book. In fact, the chairman of the company, who has far too much lush brown hair into his fifties, has deftly circumvented the hiring of top-level bald guys by naming women to run each of his divisions. Oh, hair, where is thy sting?!?

When I brought the proposal for this book to my agent, the white-maned Jay Acton, he was unenthusiastic. Naturally. He has hair. Lots of it. When he exhibited ambivalence, in extremis, I looked at him for a long moment.

"Jay," I said, breaking a short silence, "I think I need a bald agent." I explained why only a bald agent would understand my intentions, and would feel that he had a personal stake in selling my book with vim and vigor.

Jay tried to show pseudo-empathy, but of course, empathy with the bald is impossible unless you are bald.

"My hair used to be a lot thicker," he said.

"But you still have it," I said.

"It turned white when I was twenty," he said.

"What a pity," I said, without consolation. "You see, Jay, when you walk out in the street, and someone has to point you out, they say, 'He's the guy with white hair.' When they point me out, it's 'the bald guy over there.' "

"Well," said Jay, "I guess I can't relate."

After an hour of my bald soliloquy, I felt I had turned Jay around, if only partially. I knew he'd never feel for the book as Irving "Swifty" Lazar, Hollywood's greatest bald agent, might. But I was satisfied. So rather than shedding Jay for an agent sans hair, I kept him and made one last request: send the proposal only to bald editors.

"Oh, c'mon, is that necessary?" Jay asked.

"No, really, I feel that they will be the most sympathetic," I said.

Reluctantly, he said he'd do what he could. He ushered me out, and said to one of his three haired assistants, "Steve, do you know of any bald editors?"

"No," he answered, "I usually speak to them by phone and they don't sound bald on the phone."

They don't sound bald on the phone!!!!!!

I glared at Jay. "I rest my case," I said. "Antibaldness prejudice lurks in this very office. I'm going to the State Human Rights Commission."

Although at first glance, Rick Wolff, my editor at Macmillan, seems to have no hair loss, he's got a fast-growing bald spot out back. Immediately, I felt that he was a brother above the scalp. With bitterness, he talks about how some of his insensitive haired relatives have sent him an old child's toy in which you move metal filings with a magnet atop the head of a bald cartoon figure named Mr. Woolly. I used to play that game, too, when I was a haired lad. It was fun then. Now it's a cruel joke.

Rick was truly excited about the book. He said he knew many people could relate to it, because he related to it, as could the top people at Macmillan, four of whom are balding. He knew it could be a Yuppie/baby boomer book.

Soon after, Rick called to say he had purchased the book for publication. He didn't say hello. All he said was: "Rich, we usually pay more to authors with hair."

I'd like to acknowledge a few people who've helped me as I wrote more and more about having less and less.

To my legion of Bald Spotters, my ace eyes in the unhaired sky who called when they sighted great baldies or helped me name great pilgarlics of the world: Arthur Pincus, who likes to take note of how the sweat beads up on my pate on hot days; Dave Rosner, David Raskin, Paul Fichtenbaum, Pete Bavasi, John Halligan, Murray Chass, Joe Horrigan, Jay Johnstone, Fred McMane, Marty Noble, Dave Klein, Bob Wolff. Special thanks to actor Ken Howard for his enthusiasm and to my former *Newsday* colleague Brad O'Hearn, one of the first bald guys to point out antibaldness bias to me.

To my old friend Steve Austin, who went bald well before me, thanks for taking flak from the haired (including me) before the flak came flying my way.

To Rick Wolff, thank you for believing in *Bald Like Me* and for having your blossoming bald spot.

To Griffin Miller, a special person who prefers bald heads to toupeed ones, thank you for your honesty.

To my closest friends, Sara Lessley, Randy Banner and Laurie Baum, lovely women who never mention that I am bald. A special thanks to Randy's husband, Jim Estrin, whose life's desire is to take aerial photos of my pate.

To my mother, Shirley Winikoff, and my grandfather, Nathan Winnik, who passed on the baldness gene, thanks a bunch. You've both made this book necessary.

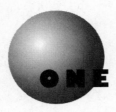

THE POWER
OF POSITIVE BALDNESS

○

The bald shall inherit the earth.
—BALDMAN

ONE WINTRY DAY I was standing on the first floor of a Manhattan office building waiting for the elevator to take me to the twenty-ninth floor. A guy with lots of dark hair stood beside me. After a few seconds of silent waiting, he turned to me and said, "I'm going for minoxidil treatments."

Now there's an attention getter. I didn't know the guy. He could have commented on the weather. But no, he wanted to tell me about the greasy potion he was rubbing into his slight bald spot. His mistake was judging my book by its bald cover and assuming I cared about him and his minoxidil. I seethed and bristled (an apt verb for us unhaired).

"Why do you think I care?" I asked.

"Well," he said, scanning my naked pate from a yard's distance, "I just figured . . ."

This was one of those rare moments when the bald can embarrass the haired.

"You know," I said, assuming my stance as the unhaired avenger, Baldman, "only 30 percent of the people who try minoxidil show any hair growth at all. What grows is nothing to crow about, either. It's like baby hair."

The guy wanted to make pleasant conversation, and got a

stern lecture instead. Maybe he generously wanted to share the hope that this dubious "cure" brought to him. Maybe he wanted to help me, lead me to a better place, where everyone has hair and everyone is happy . . .

Naaaaahhhh. He was mocking me, pitying me. I was his vision of a future he never wanted to face, the Ghost of Baldness Future; his worst unhaired nightmare. What he meant to say was this: "I've lost twelve hairs and damned if I'm going to lose twelve thousand more like you, baldie."

I continued my attack, knowing that the hearts and scalps of my bald brethren were behind me. Said I: "I hope the rest of your hair falls out—now. Have a nice day."

Men, being bald need not be the end of the line for your head. It can be a new beginning. It can be a new dawn in our lives. We can boldly accept our baldness without buckling under to the haired profiteers who seek to falsify our heads with minoxidil, hairpieces and transplanted hair plugs.

From this moment on, we can celebrate each and every bare pate—past, present and future.

We can strike back when our bald brothers are slighted by cries of "baldie," "chrome dome" and "cue ball."

We can stand tall, knowing our haircuts are cheap, our hats don't flatten our hair, our chances for dandruff are reduced. We can comb our head with a wash towel and we can truly get a full-body tan.

We can lay waste to the hair-is-better argument by questioning whether it is even normal to *have* hair!

Hair is merely a useless load of stringy protein that's gotten excessively positive hype. Hair makes us crazy and makes us jealous. Hair obsesses us and ages us. It splits, greases, oils, mats, frizzes, sticks up, sticks out, falls in our eyes when we putt and costs too much to keep.

Then what good is hair?

None.

Then—off with it all!

Be bald!
Be proud!
To paraphrase the Edwin Starr song, "War," I say:

> *Hair*
> *What is it good for?*
> *Absolutely nothing.*
> *(Say it again)*
> *Hair*
> *What is it good for?*
> *Absolutely nothing.*
> *(Say it again)*

There are so many pressures on us unhaired to be ashamed of our bare heads. The media. Advertising. Cosmetics companies. Evil hairmeisters. Ignorant people on the street. They've all conspired to make us think there's something wrong with us, that we are diseased and need to be cured of our affliction. We bald folk are the Rodney Dangerfields of the headed world. Our pates get no respect at all.

No matter what age in human history you name, there were ignorant bands of antibaldies spreading the lie that bald men are lesser men. Bald cavemen were clubbed to death by their haired colleagues. Samson cut off his hair and lost his power. Julius Caesar, balding himself, sheared the hair off Gallic prisoners as a sign of submission to Rome. And remember that Caucasian pioneer heads were stripped bare by the scalpings of American Indians, an action that is painfully symbolic.

There are accounts of aristocrats and kings so upset by their loss of hair that they took to wearing wigs. Second-century Romans even painted ersatz hair on their bald scalps. In the court of King Louis XIII, Abbé de la Rivière started sporting a long blond wig in 1620; four years later, *Le Roi de Bald* was outfitted with false hair.

Not long after, King Louis XIV, bald by nature, wore a long, black flowing wig, setting the silly style of the day. Old Louie never, ever let an outsider see him au naturel. So paranoid was he that at bedtime, he passed his wig to a servant through his drawn bed curtain; in the morning, the servant passed the pseudo-locks back the same way.

We bald guys had our defenders, even back in the Dark Ages. Saint Anselm, the archbishop of Canterbury, allowed no one in his cathedral with false or long hair. And King Henry I abolished wigs and long hair. Bald is bald, they said, that's all. No big deal. They were heroes of any age.

Unfortunately, no one has made such necessary rules stick since the twelfth century. And those guys, bless their just souls, never met today's hairmeisters, read *GQ* or watched TV, where the folly that we baldies are second-class citizens is fostered.

I long for old-fashioned vengeance, where a bald guy can inflict simple, swift punishment upon his mockers.

Take the biblical story of the prophet Elijah and his disciple Elisha traveling from Gilgal. After they had crossed the Jordan River, a flaming chariot and a team of horses took Elijah heavenward in a whirlwind, leaving Elisha alone.

On his way to Bethel, Elisha was accosted by a gang of sniveling boys who shouted at him, "Go up, baldhead! Go up, baldhead!" I'm not sure where "up" was, but you can still imagine Elisha's angry reaction to this epithet and the trumped-up importance of hair way back then. Elisha must have known his haireth was goneth, and didn't need a bunch of kids to remindeth him.

So he cursed them in the name of the Lord, whereupon two she-bears came out of the woods and tore the forty-two tykes to pieces. Believe me, they didn't live to mock a baldie again.

"Vengeance is mine," saith the Lord, who, at the time, must have been bald or had clued into the early growth of biblical baldness bias. To my dismay, He hasn't equalized things so even-handedly in a few millennia.

I don't like to admit that Baldman had ancient forefathers

because I'd prefer to think my ideas are original. But I'm forced to admit that the Spanish-born writer Martial, who trained his outrageous satirical eyes on first-century Rome, is my truest ancestor. This great deflator of hairism wrote:

> From the one side and the other, you gather up your scanty locks and you cover, Marinus, the wide expanse of your shining bald scalp with the hair from both sides of your head. But blown about, they come back at the bidding of the wind, and return to themselves, and gird your bare poll with big curls on this side and on that . . . Will you please, in simpler fashion confess yourself old, so as after all to appear a bald person. *Nothing is more unsightly than a bald man covered with hair* (italics mine).

What a brilliant condemnation of combovers—and done so wittily in Latin! Quite often now, I feel the voice of Martial channeled through me, telling the world that bald is bald and never should a false hair be placed upon it!

If Martial was not bald, I'm sure he had the soul of a bald man. I know I have had one since I was twenty-one when the hairs started tumbling and my drain started clogging. Here I was, a junior in college, and *balding!* Nothing could possibly make me feel older and less confident of myself. It's a typical reaction of the young bald. I was angry, but the nature of the anger was such that my words sounded as if I had cancer. "Why me?" I asked. "Why me?"

My family was of no help.

"You have lots of curly hair," my mother told me.

"I don't see anything different," said my stepfather.

"Uncle Richie is going bald," said my sensitive but perceptive nephew as I held him in my arms.

But I grew up. I wasn't a man until I accepted being bald. It was just folderol about becoming a man when I was bar mitzvahed at age thirteen.

I agonized.

I combed over.

I used hair spray.

I contemplated forming Baldies Anonymous. *"My name is Richard S. and I'm bald."*

So I had my hair mitzvah at about age twenty-eight, uttered a silent Blessing over the Pate ("God grant me the serenity to accept the hair I do not have . . .") and accepted it. There was no ritual. It was done. My hair was gone, fluttered up to the Big Cigar Box in the Sky. The only locks I'd have would be on bagels.

Yet I remain angry—not with being bald but at the Gang of Hairmeisters, a race worthy of a tale of their own by the Brothers Grimm. The anger put me on my current mission from the Bald God. I had to become Baldman, the Unhaired Avenger, to fight the haired enemies. I pledged myself to continue the battle for as long as it took, so that one day I'd be regarded as simply a man, and not as "the bald guy over there in the corner."

I vowed to fight on to help the Silent Baldority, those bald men who suffer in silence, those voiceless pilgarlics who have never accepted their baldness.

GUYS—THIS PATE'S FOR YOU!

At the top of my list of evil is minoxidil, the blood-pressure medicine found to (maybe) grow hair. Quick, have you ever seen a full head of minoxidil hair? No one has. It doesn't exist. Minoxidil grows sparse peach fuzz, maybe 10, maybe 20, maybe 30 percent of the time. Depends on your head. It won't work if you're a chrome dome and it shows results generally with guys who've just started losing it. It puts their baldness in a kind of holding pattern. But it ain't no miracle.

Did you see the first TV commercial for minoxidil? The Upjohn Company, a very reputable pharmaceutical company, is selling it under the Rogaine brand name. The ad is shot in pleasant hues, like douche and feminine deodorant spray commercials. It shows a good-looking guy walking alone on a beach, speaking to himself, incredulous that he, of all people, should have *thinning* hair. *Thinning!* Such problems, he has! They couldn't even get a truly *bald* guy! If minoxidil were so good they could have really proven the worth of the drug by casting a guy whose head reflects the setting sun.

At the end of the spot, this message appears: "If you have questions about baldness, speak to your doctor." Hard-hitting! Sells the product masterfully!

Upjohn's second hard-hitting commercial featured a guy with blond curly hair and a very embryonic bald spot in the back. He looks at the mirror and concludes: "I'm not bad now, but I wouldn't mind looking better."

Value judgments all over the place! To every hairmeister, bald is bad and hair is better. Why is hair thought of as better than bald? We cannot think that way. They're equals, men, not rivals.

I can think of a more truthful way to sell Rogaine. Put an

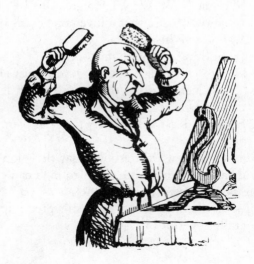

ordinary Joe in his bathroom, wearing a sleeveless T-shirt, combing his hair and looking down the sink drain to see what he's
lost.

Voice-over: Hey, baldie. Yeah, you. The chrome dome.

(Guy looks up.)

Voice-over: Have I got somethin' for you! Rogaine. Just rub
it in your head every day for the rest of your life.

(Guy has quizzical look on his face.)

Voice-over: It's kinda like the Pill. If you don't use it, you
lose it. You'll love that oily, unctuous feeling. And maybe you'll
grow some stray bits of peach fuzz.

The hairmeisters want to sell hair as *healthy* and baldness as
sick. Wrong. Wrong. Wrong. Baldness is a natural, if not always
welcome, process in the march of time. If being hirsute or bald
were options in a multiple-choice test, most of us bald guys would
choose hair. But the Great God of Hair doesn't grant us that
choice.

In a TV testimonial for the Helsinki Formula, a so-called
cure from Finland (have you ever heard a Finn complain about
being bald?), a man says, "Going bald was the *worst* thing that
ever happened to me." WOW! What a great life he's had! Imagine: losing his hair was worse that a loved one dying or a divorce
or cancer! I wanna live his life.

Baldness is nothing to be ashamed of.

It is nothing to call your doctor or psychiatrist about.

It is less consequential than the flu, a broken leg, obesity,
alcoholism, cancer or a heart attack.

In fact, baldness doesn't cause *any* physical pain. In fact, it
might be beneficial.

Women have written Dear Abby to say they don't care that
their men are bald. One beautiful soul wrote: "I can't verify that
bald men are better lovers, but my hunch is that a man who has
lost his hair—or is losing it fast and isn't preoccupied by the
fact—is generally superior in bed."

Men, we need a positive attitude about baldness. I got mine after suffering from the verbal slings of the haired.

Because I know what it's like to be driving and hear some haired yahoo scream out: "Nice car . . . Nice head."

I know how annoying it is when a relative says, "Have you considered a toupee?"

I know how it feels when a haired friend (a *friend*, no less) says, "Isn't it interesting how Rich's head sweats?"

I have heard the sound of pity from a strange woman who was pointing out the red, sunburned state of my pate during the summer. "Ooh, does it hurt?" she asked.

We must exhibit the positive attitude necessary to acquire Bald Pride. We must make peace with our pates. Part of the path is to remember these pointers:

1. Bald men have rights just like the haired, so don't accept second-class treatment. If a woman talks to your head instead of into your eyes, stare at her chest (for more bald rights, see "The Bald of Rights" later in this book). If you've been denied a job because you're bald, sue in federal court or write to me at the Baldness Anti-Defamation League.

2. Hairpieces, though they have improved technically, can be easily spotted by the trained eye. Would you rather be bald or stared at derisively as a wearer of a toupee (a word the hairmeisters detest)? You will always live in fear of it falling off or coming loose at the wrong moment (or falling into your soup if you forget to tape it down).

3. Minoxidil treatments don't work very well.

4. Hair transplants are ugly, bloody and don't always work. Even when they do, they leave you with a head that looks like a bad corn crop in Nebraska after a drought.

5. Hair weaves risk embarrassment when your real hair (to which your weave is woven) grows, causing the weave to move. Your hair will look like an image from a fun-house mirror. Weaves can also cause further baldness by their method of attachment.

6. Hair doesn't always look very good. Take a look at Don King, Cyndi Lauper and Ted Koppel. Do they benefit by having all that hair?

7. Baldness is easy. No muss. No fuss. You can increase general productivity by not worrying about your hair.

8. Baldness is a look, just as a hairstyle is. If you groom your remaining hair well and keep your dome clean, you can stand out as never before.

9. Going bald all the way to a shaved head is the path to immediate notice and sexiness (see Yul Brynner and Telly Savalas). Women will want to touch and caress your head just to see what it's like. You also seem ageless because your hair never turns gray or white.

10. Being bald and not covering up or combing over shows you are true to yourself. You're not trying to hide anything. This is the real you, take it or leave it.

O

Bald men, it's time to unite. I'd say you have nothing to lose but your hair, but you've already lost it. So don't lose your confidence to the drumbeat of the haired forces of the world. Hairism shall fall. Baldism is the way of truth, the way for the next millennium.

For we know, as Carl Reiner once said, that "the guys with hair are overdressed."

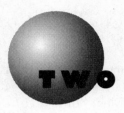

DEAR YUL:
DIARY OF A BALD MAN

○

THE HAIRMEISTERS' ADS promise hair. They're tantalizing and tonsorially titillating. Stuck in the back of newspapers along with tire sales and aired at four in the morning between commercials for tummy-tightening Abdomenizers, they share a message of faith, hope and snake-oil fakery.

They say, in their own ways, "Hey, kids, let's build some hair! Let's get rugs, plugs and drugs—and do it!"

"You're a man," says the ad for Hair Now Cosmetic Surgery, "you look in the mirror and the one thing you were proudest of—your hair—is thinning out. Will it stop? Could you adjust to a hairpiece?"

Shorter advertising hooks make similar vows, with offers of minoxidil, hairpieces and transplants. Drum roll, please. Cue up to intro of "Also Sprach Hairathustra."

(Dum)

Medical breakthrough: We can grow hair.

(Dum)

Some men get ahead by starting at the top.

(Dum-dum)

End baldness with Derma-Bond.

(Dum)

He looks great for someone who's bald.

(Dum)

Go to the top with Carmine Merlino the Magician.

(Da-Dummmmmmmm!)

And the most famous words in all of hair replacement, from the top of the hair-woven head of hairmeister Sy Sperling, owner of the Hair Club for Men: *"I'M NOT ONLY THE HAIR CLUB PRESIDENT, I'M ALSO A CLIENT."*

Even though I'm philosophically anti–hair replacement, I felt I had to give some of these places their due. I can't criticize what I don't know. What if I'm wrong? What if I'm damning them without giving them a fair chance to explain themselves? If I am truly to be Baldman—fighting for truth, justice and the hairless way—shouldn't I go head-to-head with the hairy foe? As they say, keep your friends close—but your haired enemies closer.

So I decided to go out undercover among the hairmeisters. All but one offered lengthy free consultations. So I visited them all as a potential client, and not as Baldman, their sworn adversary. I wanted to know what they could do, how they would do it, and what it would cost. I wanted to know the nature of these hairists and whether they were truly antibald.

I had to know the nature of my enemy and report back to Yul, my hairless spiritual father.

DAY 1: FIRST ENCOUNTERS OF THE HAIRED KIND

Dear Yul,

So this is what they look like, the Three Hairedmen of the Bald Apocalypse: a transplant surgeon, a representative from Upjohn and a hairpiece maker. They're here, in—get this!—the Eisenhower Room of the Long Island Marriott Hotel, for a seminar on hair replacement. Ike would have loved the irony.

The room is filled with seventy-five guys in various states of balding. One man behind me wears a black hairpiece atop gray fringe hair. Another in front sports a full-head gray piece that fits like a loose helmet. Some have too much hair to be concerned. They must be scoping out the futures market, I suppose.

This is my first encounter with the enemy. I want to heckle. I want to disrupt the conference, proclaim them frauds and walk away triumphantly. But I'm the only one here who is anti–hair replacement. Everyone else seems to *need* to be here. So I stay mum.

The leader is Gary Hitzig, a transplant surgeon who organized the seminar. He's bald by trade, had one shoddy transplant, wore a toupee, then had a better transplant that gave him a good head of hair.

He tells us:

"If you want to keep your hair, you can cut off your testicles, which is what the Italian singing group, the Castratas, did. They kept their voices high and hair on their heads."

(A joint, collective shudder goes through the audience.)

"I get fathers with full heads of hair who come in with their bald sons. They're guilty. They say, 'Did I do this to him?' " "A transplant isn't a shiatsu massage, but it's not painful. We give nitrous oxide and novocaine. If your teeth are drilled, you bleed. With this, you bleed, too."

Next up was a nervous Ernie Diamond of Upjohn, maker of minoxidil (a.k.a. Rogaine), the surprisingly unpopular bald balm that grows fuzzy little hairs on tiny bald spots. Some say it stops hair loss; others say it is of minimal aid. Ernie dances around queries about Rogaine's powers.

Diamond is nonplussed by a few tough questions. When challenged on the claims made in a video he showed, he admits: "Rogaine is not a panacea. It isn't a miracle and many people are disappointed if their expectations are too high. We don't make wild claims. For many people, stabilizing the loss and keeping it where it is is enough."

The hairpiece maker, known simply as Donte (Mr. Donte to you), is a broad-smiling, curly-haired refugee from the beauty salon world. He fairly glows about his hairpieces.

"I think synthetics are wonderful," he says, beaming. "My fabrics are wonderful fibers, wonderful fabrics."

Ah, now this is more like it. This is the moment I've been waiting for. I'm ready to pounce. Donte isn't selling hair. He's selling fabrics. Beautiful, wonderful fabrics.

Donte's not merely a hairmeister. He's an *upholsterer!*

Later, I try to corner Diamond but he's nowhere to be found. So I seek out Donte, who offered the men a chance to see themselves in a selection of hairpieces. Donte is excited. Fabrics are his life and he likes to show off. He's peeling a piece off a young, brown-haired baldie (he doesn't look half-bad) when I ask him to give my head a whirl.

Out from his red satchel—not much different from a gym bag in appearance and scent—comes a bouffant salt-and-pepper piece that looks as big as my head. It's scary. *This is gonna go on my head?!?* It's so . . . Abbie Hoffman.

"Come, sit over here," says Donte, using the tone of a happy-go-lucky dentist. He plunks the synthetic monster (so much like a rug that I think a shag is being laid on my pate) on me and starts combing with a fake hair-filled brush. On my head, it feels as odd as it looks. I raise my hand to feel the fabric. I'm a wood floor being carpeted, a La-Z-Boy being reupholstered.

A crowd gathers around us. They watch with interest. It's quiet with anticipation, like a crowd watching Jack Nicklaus putt.

"Oooh, it's lovely," says Donte.

"Do you have a mirror?" I ask.

"No," he says. Some hairdresser. Two women donate their makeup compacts, so I try to gauge my look through two tiny round mirrors. It's not that easy. But I see enough.

Good Lord, I have a hairline! Good Lord, I look absurd! A salt-and-pepper soufflé tops my brown curls. My scalp is unaccustomed to this. It's having an epiphany. Am I hallucinating? Is it real or is it fabric? I haven't had a hair—real or wonderful synthetic—on my head in ten years.

Donte smiles as I angle the compacts for the best view.

"You look wonderful," he says.

"Just like your beautiful fabric," I say.

DAY 2: OOH, YOUR LOSS IS REALLY BAD

Dear Yul,

The seminar was a big step. But sitting down to consult with a hairmeister means more—it means that I might be persuaded of the rightness of hair replacement. Will I be swayed? Will I suffer from the Stockholm Hostage Syndrome, where I start identifying with my haired captors?

My first stop is Men's Hair Now, where hairpieces are attached to bald heads, with some sort of super-secret medical emulsion. That's glue, to you and me.

"Do you think I can grow hair?" is the first thing owner Michelle Cipriano says to me.

(I don't know, I think, can you squeeze hard enough?)

"No," I reply, "I know you can't."

"What do you know about male pattern baldness?"

"That I have it," I explained.

(Is a pop quiz the first rite of hair replacement?)

She peers at me. She's pleasant but she has an urgent edge, as if she has a quota of male tundras to fill that day.

"So you must be bald for twenty years, right?" she says.

"Wrong," I answer, my ire rising, "I wasn't bald at twelve. I can assure you I had plenty of hair then."

"Well, you were probably losing it for five years before you noticed it," she says, not missing a beat.

"That would have made me seventeen when my baldness began."

"Oh, okay."

She shows me a looseleaf binder filled with her before-and-after photos. A lot of the before pictures show men with hairlines

like mine, but every time she talks about each man, she looks
at my head and says:

"But his loss isn't as bad as yours," or,

"You're a little worse than this one," or,

"Your hair loss is really bad."

So I'm being confronted with moral and qualitative judgments about my hair loss. Bald is bad. Bald is worse (than hair).

When she leaves her office for a moment I notice, leaning
on a wall, a frame containing several photographs. The frame is
not hung on the wall because Men's Hair Now—such an im-
perative, isn't it?—just moved from several blocks away.

The frame has two photos of bad hair weaves, but they're
harmless. Ugly but harmless. What stand out are two color shots
of a man in mid-transplant. Blood is everywhere, even on the
frame, I think. I wonder if the man died. The poor guy looks
like boxer Chuck "The Bayonne Bleeder" Wepner after being
mauled by Muhammad Ali.

Is this a selling point? Is she a negative campaigner in the
race for voters' pates? "I promise not to turn you bloody!" could
be her campaign slogan.

"I used to do transplants," Michelle says, "and I used to do
weaves. I stopped when I developed Perma-Bond." She pronounces it matter-of-factly, as if she'd hypothesized the Big Bang
Theory for the first time.

As we talk, she spots a customer waiting for a consultation
and tut-tuts. "Look at him," she says, "such a bad weave. He
looks awful. I get a lot of people like that. I have to fix up other
people's work."

She tells me Perma-Bond is similar to what dentists use to
bond teeth. The glue—Krazy Glue for the head, so to speak—
is applied to the periphery of the bald area, dissolves into the
scalp but retains the bond. Every four to six weeks, you must
return for a lube job that includes removal of the piece with a
solvent that releases the bond.

Michelle unwraps curly brown hair, like mine, from around

a tiny spindle, combs it out and beckons me to follow her to a styling alcove. Now she takes the little curls and places them on my head. They cover very little but she is exultant.

"What a difference!" she exclaims.

(Well, not really. I now have a thimbleful of hair on my head, which covers as much space as a sprig of parsley.)

"Well, it's hard to tell," I say.

"I guess I'd need more hair," she says, "because you have such a big forehead."

("My, what a big forehead you have, Grandma!")

("The better to go bald on, my dear!")

"We'll need more hair falling onto your forehead because you have such a long face," she adds.

So let's sum up. According to Michelle, I have:

1. a long face;
2. a really bad hair loss;
3. a huge forehead;
4. been bald since age twelve.

I tell her I want to shop around, which angers her, a reaction that reinforces my belief that hairmeisters are venal folks to be avoided like Jim and Tammy Faye Bakker.

"What do you think you'll find?"

"I don't know," I say, "but I'm just starting to look."

"You won't find anything better."

"Maybe, but the worst thing you can do is a hard sell."

"I wouldn't think of it," she says, "but you'll be back. Remember, nobody will do what I did. Nobody else will show you examples of the hair we use and our customers. They'll just show you a video and a couple of pictures."

My first date with a hairmeister is a total disaster, and I'm ecstatic, Yul. She fulfills all the stereotypes I was looking for and didn't persuade me to cover my head.

DAY 3: I'VE DONE FIFTEEN HAIRPIECES
FOR BURT REYNOLDS

Dear Yul,

As I wait a half-hour for Top Priority owner Harvey Russo to wait on me, I bide my time with my talisman, a biography of Winston Churchill. I read about the greatest political baldie of the twentieth century so I have the inner fortitude to remember my simple equation: Baldness equals greatness. Again: Baldness equals greatness. Winnie is my grip on the bald reality and I carry him with me to all hairmeister calls.

Russo's place is in a corner of an aging industrial building on Fifth Avenue and could use a paint job and nice carpeting. But Harve, himself, makes up for what his place lacks. He's a short, lithe, friendly guy with flowing gray hair topped by one of his own hairpieces. I can't tell where the piece starts and his real hair begins. Judging by the photographs on his wall of Harvey

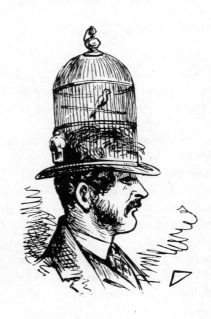

and Willard Scott, it appears old Harve has had to color his piece quite a lot in the past few years to keep up with his aging side hairs.

We talk inside a styling booth, complete with a sink, combs, brushes and Barbasol.

"My friends say they don't remember me losing my hair," Harvey says. "I did it gradually, the best way. I didn't want to be as bald as you are."

(A little needle to my scalp, but not too bad.)

Harve and I talk hair, real and synthetic, how he sews hair onto a variety of lightweight bases and Burt Reynolds. Burt, of course, doesn't admit his baldness even though any astute Burt-watcher would know of his baldness since the late 1960s. Burt and Frank Sinatra are Hairpiece Moguls, men who won't admit their hairlessness, but Hollywood rumor has it they both have at least twenty hairpieces apiece.

"I do Burt Reynolds and Willard Scott," says Harvey. I wonder if he's leaking a big secret and word of this breach will cut him off as Burt's nonexclusive rug man. "I've done about fifteen pieces for Burt. I was just down at his house in Florida. What a place"—the House that Hairpieces Built.

"I see that Burt's got a gray one now," I say.

"Well, it was about time," Harve says.

As for Sinatra, Harve's only got hairpiece grapevine poop: "His weave fell out and now he's back to pieces."

I wonder who does Frank's pieces?

Harvey and I talk about hair brokers, a subject I first learned about with Michelle at Men's Hair Now. When hairmeisters need hair for a piece, they have to get it from somewhere. They need virgin—unbleached, unpermed and so forth—from places like India, Europe and Asia, not violated hair from the United States.

Turns out there really are hair middlemen who go around to poor areas and pay women (only women) to sell them hair which they've cut off from the center of their heads, which accounts for the prevalence of hair buns in poverty-pockets of Italy, India and Korea.

Harve holds a spindleful of brown curly hair like my own. "I'll say to a middleman, 'Get me some of this,' " and back from Italy it'll come. What flabbergasts me is the price. An ounce of my kind of hair would go for $240 an ounce. If I'd known it was so valuable, I'd have saved it and sold it back to myself at a discount.

"It's cheaper to buy lox," I say.

"And tastier," says Harve.

Harve likes my hair, what's left of it. It's curly, bouncy and easy to blend with a curly haired hairpiece.

"I like to make my pieces look easy and loose," he says, "the looser the better and the easier it is to make it look natural.

"I have to know a lot about you," he continues. "How active you are in sports and in the sack. I adjust it to your lifestyle. You may have to blend in synthetic with some real hair."

Synthetic hair lasts longer than real hair. Real hair is dead hair the minute Concetta snips hers off and saves it for the hairbroker in Palermo. While it doesn't turn gray, it isn't being fed nutrients. It looks good for a while, but it oxidizes in the air (that is, turns red and yellow with too much exposure), and lasts, with regular wear, maybe twelve or eighteen months. Synthetic hair feels like a hairbrush, but it's sturdy and lasts longer. It's also cheaper and doesn't require cutting off Concetta's beautiful dark-brown locks.

"Monsanto makes synthetic hair," says Harve. "It's not real hair, but it's better than what's been out there before."

Now that's something Monsanto doesn't say much about. Monsanto, the maker of AstroTurf, makes HairTurf. I have to assume that a head full of HairTurf will drain quickly in the rain but will cause all sorts of knee problems for people running on my head. I think I'd prefer real hair.

Now Harve's trying a brown, slightly pompadoured hairpiece on me. He attaches it with double-backed tape and combs it into my head frame. It looks natural. It looks, I shudder to say, good. I really hate to say it, but I like Harve and I like the hairpiece.

I think I'm starting, slightly, to lose a grip on being Baldman. I could do *this,* I think to myself. No, you can't, I reply. Yes, I can, I retort.

I move my head from angle to angle. Harve gives me a big mirror to view it from the back. From the back! Hair in the back! Say Hallelujah! My own hairstylist knows never to lift a mirror to the back of my head. I know what's not there.

But this! My head is filled with an ounce of Italian hair! And I look . . . well, like a bald man. No matter how much hair I appear to have, I still look bald. I see the hair but I don't. The hair seems only to serve as a frame for my bald head. It's like the stories you hear about amputees who still sense the nerves and muscles of their old legs and reach out in the middle of the night to scratch an itch on their thigh, only to find nothing there. I feel that way, too. I see hair, but it's a mirage. I see a bald head. Hairpiece or not, I'm still a bald man. The voices in my head are battling, and the bald one is winning.

Harve tells me a rug like the one on my head costs about $1,600. A similar synthetic one would go for $1,200.

"When you walk down the street," I ask, "can you spot any hairpiece?"

"Any one," he says. "It's my business. It's an instinct. We all have certain talents. If I can't spot them, I'm in trouble. I can sense them no matter how good they are." Must be a recessive toupee-spotting gene.

Even though I've fought off some of the hairpiece-looks-good demons, I'm still torn. I call my editor, Rick, to tell him the most salient point of my investigation of the day.

Rick: Hello . . . Rick Wolff here.

Me: Baldman here.

Rick: What's happening, Baldman?

Me: You won't believe it. I just met Burt Reynolds's toupeemaker. What an honor.

Rick: Really. You're sure uncovering things.
Me: So to speak.

DAY 4: HERE, FEEL MY HEAD

Dear Yul,
International Hair Design, a few blocks from Harvey's place, is in a recently restored townhouse. It's a slick place, run by Stella Neste, an ex-manager of Sy Sperling's Hair Club for Men. She left Sy after fifteen years when he started using Korean hair for his pieces.

"Stelllllaaaaaaa!" I can hear Sy scream. "I'm gonna use Korean hair."

"No, Sy, darlin'," Stella replies, "don't y'all know it's got too much kim chee in it?"

So in leaving—a departure that pained Sy—she brought in investors and opened IHD, where, instead of Sy's Strand-by-Strand system, she uses the Inter-Strand system. Big deal: it means they sew each hair into a base one by one. After the hairs (European only) are sewn to a base, a braid of nylon fiber is woven across the great expanse of a bald spot, to which the Inter-Stranded piece is attached.

I am waiting to be called in for a consultation when a burly guy named John, wearing a casual black and silver ensemble, greets me. He's got short dark hair that at first glance looks like his own. He chats me up, so I think he's waiting for an appointment, too. He sounds like a dockworker. But he is, in actuality, a rug representative.

"Come into the office," he says after pleasantries.

John leads me into a luxurious office with a gray motif. There's a TV console and a VCR and a couple of couches. He looks at me from behind his too-small black desk and pronounces me a perfect IHD customer: "Curly hair. You'll look great."

John tells me the story of his hair. He went bald young and

wore a hairpiece. A few years ago, he had a transplant that failed him, but he doesn't blame the transplant doc. "We're still friends," he says sincerely. Then he came in for a weave from Stella.

"She left Sy Sperling a year ago and we've taken away a lot of his customers," says John.

This is the goal for some hairmeisters: kidnap Sy's baldies and make them their own. There seems to be a growing trade in the Sperling market from all kinds of hairmeisters. Pretty soon, the Chicago Board of Options will have a big trade in Sperling Woven Hair Futures.

"We're spending $1 million on commercials and print ads," says John, "and if you buy this in the next month, we'll give it to you for $1,500, not the normal $3,000. We've got a lot of people who normally go to Sperling."

There it is again. Poor Sy. If this goes on, the Hair Club could be merely the Hair Kaffeeklatsch for Men.

John shows me the new TV commercial that will run in the wee hours when bald men are emotionally weak and tonsorially susceptible. Immediately, I see this pseudo-hair emporium's attitude toward bald men: in the commercial, a bald man stops his sportscar to ask: "What's wrong with this picture?"

Again, baldness is viewed as *wrong*. How can anyone make right or wrong judgments about baldness?

I ask John a standard question: Can I see a Neste hairpiece? He leaves the room for a moment, and I hear Stella say, "Everything is custom-made."

John returns to say there are no hair spares, "but would you like to touch my head?"

I walk over, feel his head, and feel the braid beneath the hair. Despite his insistence that "it's undetectable," close examination reveals that it is detectable. Not bad. But detectable. But I don't want to quash his ardor so I stay quiet. He's also much larger than I am.

I ask John about the Inter-Strand system. Isn't that the same as Sy Sperling's system and other similar weaves?

"Yes," he says, sputtering, "but we do it better."

When I come home, my answering machine reveals hair-meister pay dirt. It's Sy Sperling, majordomo of the Hair Club. "Please call back as soon as you can, Richard," I hear, "about the interview you want to do with me."

I can't wait. The excitement of meeting a man who is both president and client leaves me all agog.

DAY 5: NOW YOU'RE A HANDSOME DEVIL

Dear Yul,

Louis looks at my head pitifully, as if to say, "Alas! Poor Yorick, I knew his hair."

Instead, Louis says, "Why did you wait so long to come to me?" (It's not as if I ignored cancer, I think, is it?)

"I don't know," I say.

"And just like that! You come in?"

Louis and I are in a minisalon with swatches of hair hanging from hooks, boxes of ready-to-wear hairpieces and wigs stacked in boxes while other pieces hang higgledy-piggledy on shelves and numerous samples of rug foundations. This must be Hair-meister Heaven.

Louis is gray-haired (his own) and middle-aged with a small potbelly. He says he's been in this business longer than he cares to think about. I'd say at least twenty-five years.

He spots a bulky, synthetic black hairpiece and plops it on my head. He turns the salon chair away from the mirror as he combs the piece into my head.

"I like a little show biz," he says, explaining that he wants to turn me around when he's done to unveil the transformation. After ten minutes of styling, it's Show Time.

"Now," he says, "you look like a handsome devil."

"That assumes I wasn't before."

"Ah, but you're truly handsome now."

"That's not what my mother would say."

The piece is neither my color nor my style. It's wavy but bulky. But still, he thinks I'm handsome.

"This is probably what you looked like . . ." he says.

". . . when I had hair?" I help him finish his thought.

"Yes."

(Well, no, I never had a dead rat on my head, Louis.)

"With the right color," Louis adds, "you can look—" and he makes a kiss accentuated by pressing two fingers into his lips and then releasing the digits quickly, as a French pastry chef might do upon seeing a perfect Napoleon.

Louis talks about his craft: "Sometimes I'm like a carpet layer. I cut out the mold of your head and lay down the carpet." (What an impressive statement of art!)

And about the origin of his pieces' hair: "It's Korean hair. But it's European quality." Is that possible?

And about spotting a forehead's old hairline: "We make you scrunch up your eyes so we can see where it used to be." (Must be like hieroglyphics.)

Louis says he can make me a piece for $1,000 that would cost me $2,500 elsewhere. "We don't have their overhead or their advertising," he says of his competitors. "We do what they do, just cheaper."

It's time to go and Louis has to remove the rug. Pulling it off is like taking a sticky Band-Aid off a stubborn scab. It hurts. Imagine the joy of having it on all day.

"I think," Louis says, "you'll be back."

DAY 6. GOOD CARS, GOOD HAIRPIECES

Dear Yul,

The Japanese are notoriously antibald. Famous bald Japanese, save Pat Morita, are hard to find. Japan happens to be the world's largest producer of hairpieces, capitalizing venally on a male population so vain that reports indicate that they are ashamed of being hairless. Ever see a bald sumo wrestler? No, they always have one of those cute little buns atop their heads.

In one article, a thirty-six-year-old Japanese man said, "I never would have been able to marry as well as I did if I had gone to the O-miai (first meeting with a prospective spouse in an arranged marriage) with a bald head."

Aderans is the biggest Japanese rugmaker and when it bought the largest United States carpetlayer in 1987, it became the world's largest of its kind. It's got a huge phony follicle factory in Japan and another big one in Thailand.

The Aderans in Manhattan looks like a doctor's office. Quickly, I meet Akinori Takai, who wears a green doctor's coat. His card informs me that he is not only the sales manager but also the head of research and development. This was a big man in fake hair!

Takai-san is a young, handsome, haired Japanese who doesn't speak English very well.

"Japanese men are bald in same percentage as American men," he tells me, "but are very shy about it. So our advertisements give only advice."

He talks about the 146 Aderans stores around the world and the beauties of mass hairpiece production.

"See, Japanese cars are made well, and so we make hairpieces well. We have big factory—big assembly line of women making hairpieces. Women have very delicate hands. We make so many pieces so that our prices moderate."

He explains the advantage of putting my scalp in the care of a big company like Aderans.

"There are no other companies that are big public companies that you can buy stock in," he says. "We are traded on Tokyo Stock Exchange. You can buy stock in us." Hmm . . . stock in locks?

Now we get down to hair and the factors that would wear down a natural-hair hairpiece.

"You swim?" he asks.

"No."

"You dive?"

"No."

"Jog?"

"No. Couch potato."

"Oily hair?"

"Yes."

"Piece will last you two years."

Takai-san doesn't have a spare piece to show me, but recommends that I not use double-backed tape.

"Use crips."

"Crips?"

"Crips," and he shows me big clips that would attach the assembly-line hair to mine.

"Oh . . . clips!"

"Yes, crips."

Cripes.

DAY 7. THE GLUE'S THE THING—BUT IT'S A BIG, BIG SECRET!

Dear Yul,

I'll say one thing for Bioexcell. They have the best hairmeister ads. Two memorable slogans say, "He Looks Great for Someone Who's Bald" and "Institute for Atrocious Hairpieces." They're pretty savvy, but having better ads than other hairmeisters is easy. Most are of dreadful, back-of-the-comic-book quality.

During my talk with Debbie of Bioexcell, I am trying to understand why a hairpiece glued on by her will cost me $2,500 while a hairpiece taped on by others will cost me from $900 to $1,600.

She says the artistry of their hairpieces and lightweight foundations are superior to their competitors', but the difference is really in the glue.

"It's the permanence," says Debbie, who looks to be in her late thirties, admits that she dyes her hair black from gray and has a schoolmarmish way about her. "Do you want to take it off and put it on like false teeth? What we give you with the permanence is something unquantifiable."

(But it *is* quantifiable. It adds up to about $1,000.)

"So you're saying the difference is the glue?" I ask.

"You'll never know how it feels until you try it," she replies, skirting my inquiry. Clearly, the higher price is driven by overhead and advertising costs. It also has a fancy, New Age name like Bioexcell to live up to, not some tacky name with Hair in it.

Nevertheless, she has not convinced me that a hairpiece she makes is so different from an artistic tape-it-on hairmeister's that it merits so much more money.

Paul, a customer turned Bioexcell salesman, comes in to show off his piece.

"People who see me regularly think I've gotten a different kind of haircut," says the walking advertisement. "I'm one of those people who always complained about losing my hair. For a long time, my family said I looked good, that it didn't matter. But I kept complaining and my mother said, 'Do something already.' "

As with other glue-it-on hairmeisters, Bioexcell customers have to return every six weeks to have the hair removed and serviced and the scalp treated.

"When they take it off," Paul continues, "you'll say, 'Did I used to look like that?' "

Paul leaves and Debbie starts the hard sell. I tell her that I still want to shop around and that I'm not yet sure what I really want to cover my head with—if I want to cover it at all.

"Why are you making this such a big decision?" she asks,

with slight irritation in her voice. "This should be an innocuous thing, not a big deal. It's not surgery.

"What are you waiting for?" she continues, now sounding exasperated after she has talked to me for thirty minutes and I have refused to sign up for hairpiece hell. "Why do you want to shop more? For what? Don't you know what you want?

"What if I took the risk out of it and promised to give you your money back on the day we put the piece on?"

"Well, I don't know," I say.

"But I can only offer it if you're ready to go ahead today."

"No, I'm not ready."

I half expect her to toss me out. I'd wasted a half-hour of her life and hadn't signed up for my glued future. She shakes my hand limply and looks at me, knowing she'll never see me again.

DAY 8. THEY TOOK A POLAROID SHOT OF MY SCALP!

Dear Yul,

I'll admit that being bald has made me camera-shy. I look better face forward, not in profile. So when Gerry Murphy, assistant to hairman Robert Cattani, tells me to pose for a Polaroid shot, I look at him and smile.

"No, bend your head forward," he says. He wants to shoot my pate, not my face! In sixty seconds, the first-ever photograph exclusively of my bald spot forms in living color.

Cattani enters soon and leads me into his office. I sit in an examining chair and he draws in green ink on the photo. He draws versions of where he'd cut into my scalp for scalp reductions—actual bloody surgical removal of skin in the bald area—that would pare down my bald expanse.

"I'd say you'll need three scalp reductions and three to four hundred hair plugs to fill your bald area," says Cattani, well-dressed, fully haired and middle-aged.

Let's add this up:

- Four reductions at $900 apiece. That's $3,600.
- Four hundred plugs at $25 per. That's $10,000.
- Only $13,600! What a bargain!

Cattani takes the green pen and starts drawing on my head. This is like kindergarten fingerpainting!

"This is one hairline," he says, then erases the ink.

He draws again.

"And this is another," he says, erasing again.

I can't tell the difference between them.

"You have a long face," he says, "so you need a prominent hairline."

I ask him about the claim in his literature that every plug he plants yields a lush harvest of hair.

"You might say a 90 percent take rate is good and that 95 percent is better," he explains, "but I guarantee 98 to 100 percent. And when I say 98 percent, I mean 100 percent. If I put ten hairs in a plug, ten will grow, not nine."

I ask him how much hair transplants contribute to his practice.

"Forty percent," he says, "but it's not growing as quickly as liposuction." For the surgically uninformed, liposuction sucks the fat out of diet- and exercise-resistant areas like women's thighs and men's love handles.

But liposuction really isn't much different from transplanting. In the haired procedure, the doctor sucks out plugs and replants them. The big difference is when the fat is sucked out, they throw it away (or maybe inject it into a genetically skinny person).

Cattani shows me slides of his successes. It reminds me of the Jackie Vernon routine where he deadpans an invisible slide show of his family on summer vacation.

"This guy," says Cattani as the first slide flashes onto a white wall, "is in his seventies and was bald, but he had perfect hair for a transplant."

The after-slide: "Now, a full head of hair."

Second mug shot: "This guy, a professional athlete in his twenties. His life was women, wine and women. Did I mention women? Naturally he was very upset he lost his hair." After-slide: "So here, we did this."

And on and on.

I ask him about the pain and healing process and side effects and he pooh-poohs them all. Of course he does. He's got a full head of hair.

Goodbye, Dr. Hair, I'll buy a Volvo with the $13,600!

DAY 9. HOWARD COSELL TAKES POOR CARE OF HIS TOUPEE

Dear Yul,

On the same floor where I found hairpiece-maker Universal Winners I discover the offices of Eva Gabor International. Besides being sister to Zsa Zsa the Traffic Criminal, Eva's role as wigmistress is even more important than her others as Merv Griffin's babe and Lisa Douglas, close friend of Arnold the Pig, Eb and Mr. Haney on *Green Acres*.

Universal is a shabby-looking place with a good reputation, left behind by its late owner, Ben Kaplan. My chef du hair, Howard, admits to wearing a full-head, dark-red hairpiece that I found only passable.

Howard is a hairpiece yenta, not unlike many a beautician, talking easily about the famous hairless.

"Burt Reynolds has very little hair. He wears a full-head piece."

"I saw Charlton Heston with a hairpiece that makes you wonder how he could walk outside with it."

"With the right makeup and special foundation, you can barely tell William Shatner wears one."

"The guy next to me does Howard Cosell's hairpieces," Howard says, in a kind of haired hush. "But Howard doesn't take care of them. They look terrible. He doesn't replace them soon enough and they turn a different color from what's left of his real hair. And he's on TV! What kind of image does he want to convey?"

Howard tells me a trick of the trade after I tell him that I'd met Reynolds's piecemaker.

"Oh, he says he makes Burt's hairpieces, huh?" Howard says. "Well, you know a lot of movie stars have their pieces made by the hairdressers on the movie sets. They're made especially for the movie and if they like them, they keep them and sometimes have more made."

As long as Howard's talkative, I also mention my visit to Bioexcell where, I tell him, they said they made their pieces in the United States.

"That's what they said?" he says. "I've seen the business they do in the same factory in Korea where we make our hairpieces."

Howard tells me he can glue his hairpieces onto my scalp exactly the way Bioexcell does—for a lot less.

"We don't have their costs," he says. "You know there's a street vendor on Thirty-ninth and Fifth who makes Chinese food. Every lunch hour, there's a long line. You have to wait an hour to get the same food they make in a restaurant for twice the price. That's how it is here. Our quality is very close. It's a matter of my artistry against theirs."

As for how Howard's sample hairpiece looks on my head— not bad. A little too gray. A little too bouffy. But not bad. There was too much hair on this piece, and it took longer to blend into my crown than I ever took to comb my hair when I had hair.

Howard notes that when a hairpiece goes blowin' in the wind, not a man will turn his head.

"You want your piece to blow in the wind," he says. "Real hair does. You want this to blow, but to blow naturally."

I agree. It blows.

DAY 10. BATMAN ... BALDMAN

Dear Yul,

I have another appointment but I cancel it when I see the window of the storefront of Edith Imre. There are a bunch of women's wigs. If I wanted a woman's wig, I'd have gone to Hooterville to see Eva Gabor.

With a few hours to kill, I decide to see *Batman*.

Instead of watching the story intently, I watch Michael Keaton. I recall from previous movies that Michael Keaton seemed to be losing lots of hair. The Michael Keaton playing Bruce Wayne–Batman has a full head of it. Not bad for a hairpiece, I think. Not bad.

Then I watch Jack Nicholson. His hair's been receding for years. Except for an appearance on the *Andy Griffith Show* in the early 1960s, I can't remember Jack without a large recession. But as the Joker, Jack has less recession than I've seen in a while. Is he augmenting that recession or is it just the angle? I wonder. I also wonder if I'm the only one in the theater wondering this.

I'm losing my grip on reality.

DAY 11. YOU CAN'T HAVE A TRANSPLANT

Dear Yul,

Mr. Quinn is blunt. He's been with the Thomas Clinics, which does transplants and other hair care work, since the end of World War II. He's sixty-nine and has a lot of gray hair. He's not a doctor but he could play one on television.

"What would you like us to do for you?" he asks.

"Well, what do you do?" I answer.

"Transplants."

He examines my head with what look like chopsticks.

"You don't have enough of a donor area. The back of your head will look like a mess if we do it," he concludes emphatically.

"So there's not much else you can do for me?"

"No. I don't want to sell you on something that won't work for you. We also ran some tests on minoxidil three years ago. We tested it for twenty months, but in most cases it didn't even stop the loss of hair."

"Is that it?" I ask.

"That's it," says Mr. Quinn.

I like that. No sales pitch. No lies. Mr. Quinn, an executive of an enemy field, is not an enemy of the people.

Bravo, Quinn.

DAY 12. BLAME IT ALL ON TONY BENNETT

Dear Yul,

The words came out very slowly.

"You definitely have . . ." says Jerry Roman, general manager of the Louis Feder hairpiece kingdom.

". . . a bald head," I say.

Jerry, a suave, gray-hairpieced man in his fifties, has a smooth way of insulting me. He's low-keyed and calm. But he's as cutting as he is cool.

"There's no reason for you to look like this." (Thank you, I say to myself, but this is the way I look, dammit!)

"You're young. God intended you to have hair. Hair frames your head. You're nice-looking and a loss of hair makes your features hard. It changes the proportions of your facial features." (You mean my nose looks even bigger hairless? Well at least I have hair in my nose!)

"Hair softens your features, makes you look your age. Being

bald makes you look older. You're a good-looking [you rake, you], casual guy; you should enhance it."

He puts a mirror up to the side of my bewigged head. This is the best hairpiece I have had on my noggin.

"See how it softens your profile?" he asks.

I can see. Yes, I can see.

Jerry espouses the Garment Theory of Hairpieces.

"You wear a hairpiece like a garment," he says. "You put your clothes on every day, you put your hairpiece on every day. You don't sleep in your clothes, do you? If you're active in bed, with a companion, you keep it on. Otherwise, you can take it off. When you wake up in the morning, you put your shirt and pants on, and you put your hairpiece on."

Jerry has a point—unless the garment on my head is a hairpiece made out of a polyester leisure suit.

After twenty-five years on the hairpiece beat, Jerry has a view of the psychology of the bald who seek a cover-up.

"When younger guys lose their hair, they're very upset," he says. "It affects their opinion of themselves, so there's a loss of confidence. Once the hairpiece is on, and he's done something about it, he regains his confidence. It's the Samson Syndrome: you regain your strength."

And Jerry's got his own Made in America view:

"The Orient may make fine computers and they may challenge Detroit in automotive expertise," Jerry says in a promotional tape he sold me for $29.95, "but when it comes to a hairpiece, for an American, worn by an American, in America, it must be made in America, by Americans."

Hallelujah! Jerry's the Lee Iacocca of ersatz hair.

I tell Jerry that I'd seen an article in which he reveals himself as a hairmeister to Frank Sinatra. He answers quietly that he is, and offers to show me the pattern from which he made a recent rug for Francis Albert. When he can't find the pattern, he brings out a current copy of *Vanity Fair* magazine and opens it to a Revlon ad featuring Frank and Barbara Sinatra.

"This is mine," Jerry says, pointing to Frank's hair, and "this is mine," gesturing to Barbara's wig.

"I finished this hairpiece for Frank in Beverly Hills," he continues. "Frank has many pieces. Of course, he doesn't admit to it. This piece gives him a squared-off look, as opposed to the Caesar look he usually wears."

As with Frank, Jerry wants a "long-term relationship" with me, if I decide on a cover-up. I don't want to fall in love, Jerry—I'm just thinking hairpiece.

Jerry's a pretty good expert on the history of fake hair. And believe it or not, he says the popularity of toupees (actually a dirty word to hairmeisters, who say it conjures up images of rugs falling into soup bowls in Three Stooges films) in recent times can be traced to a 1954 article in *Life* magazine that featured old Louis Feder and revealed that the teen heartthrob of the moment, singer Tony Bennett, wore a toupee.

So now I can definitively affix blame. It's Tony Bennett's fault. Thank you, Jerry. My search has ended.

DAY 13. ABOUT AS STRONG AS KRAZY GLUE

Dear Yul,

Today I learned a new word.

Quinnoidal.

That's the name of the glued-on hairpiece made by the Penthouse for Men, a fancy rug emporium.

My hyperactive stylist-salesman, Patrick, explained a quinnoidal as the invention of his partner, to connote, in a way, a scientific term for a compound with double bonding.

Great marketing term. Quinnoidal. One of the few words it rhymes with is hemorrhoidal. The slogan possibilities are endless.

Pat is very excited about this glued-on quinnoidal. The Penthouse, he says, spent "eight f——g months" with a chemical company testing the glue used to apply it.

"I guarantee it's three times stronger than what Bioexcell uses," he says. "We wanted to make it as strong as Krazy Glue. We came close, but we can't guarantee that you can stick to a building girder and hang off it like they do in the Krazy Glue commercial."

I am disappointed. I had hoped to wear my quinnoidal on the thirty-eighth floor of the frame of a skyscraper.

"When Elliott, my partner, went to Boca wearing his quinnoidal, he called me four times a day, telling me, 'I dove with it,' 'I showered with it,' 'I swam with it and it didn't come off!' For him to say that is something because he's one tough f——g cookie."

Pat has a theory just the reverse of Jerry Roman's. He insists that the quinnoidal should never be treated as a mere garment, but a semipermanent piece of you.

"You don't really want to take it off. Do you say to a lover, 'You put your things in the drawer and I'll put my hair on this mannequin's head'? That may bother you. Some guys don't want to wake up in the morning and see their bald selves. They like the way they look with hair and don't want to stop."

Quinnoidal. That'll go up there with another word I've learned in my travels: the hinkle. A hinkle was supposedly named for a vain German general with a combover that from above looked like a tornado funnel. Imagine the chuckles enemy soldiers had when they saw his ridiculous swirl. Or just imagine what his colleagues might have said.

"Ach, Herr Hinkle, you look like a putz!"

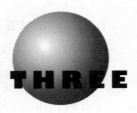

THREE

HE'S NOT ONLY THE PRESIDENT
OF THE HAIR CLUB FOR MEN . . .

O

HE'S NOT ONLY A CLIENT . . .
HE'S AN ENEMY OF THE PEOPLE!
—MY INTERVIEW WITH SY SPERLING

THE BEST-KNOWN PERSON in the hair replacement world is late. The waiting area is empty except for the haired receptionist and me. When Sy arrives, fifteen minutes after our appointed meeting time, he steps out of the elevator schlepping two shopping bags full of clothes. Quickly, he darts to and from several offices in the Hair Club for Men suite, singing "Let's Spend the Night Together." He had listened to the Rolling Stones on the way in and can't get them out of his head. "You like Mick Jagger?" he asks me.

In person, Sy is not entirely the uncomfortable-looking man you see in his infamous low-rent, late-night Hair Club commercials. He is taller than I expected, about six-foot-four, and looks younger than his forty-eight years.

His hair, of course, is perfectly coiffed. Hang around him for a month or two and you'll see that it never grows—a sure sign of a hairpiece. Either that, or amazing willpower.

When he opens his mouth, Hair Club Sy emerges in his full pseudo-haired glory: this is the man who has covered twenty thousand heads with his woven-to-your-hair-with-nylon-filament pieces and assaults us with ads for the company he created with his wife, Amy, in 1968. Wherever you are in this land of ours (for Hair Clubs are growing apace, like Lady Godiva's hair), you may have seen the ads, starring Sy and his grating Bronx accent.

"I'm not only the president of the Hair Club for Men," he says with nary a trace of emotion, "I'm a client."

Sy *has* to be for real; nobody would go out and purposely hire a spokesman so stiff that he makes Ralph Kramden as the Chef of the Future on *The Honeymooners* look as smooth as Ricardo Montalban pitching rich Corinthian leather.

Even the Hair Club minions know a little camp when they see it. They know the image—which Sy describes as being more credible than having a celebrity spokesman—Sy projects. While I am there, they show Sy a new corporate brochure in which one page has a headline asking, "Is There Really a Sy Sperling?"

Yes, there is, as sure as there is a Santa Claus. Sometimes I didn't know if he was truly for real, but I can tell you that he exists, much as you and I do. The biggest exception is that he has a poor Indian woman's hair sitting on his bald scalp, colored to match his natural hair and baked in a special oven (kids, don't try this at home!) to mold the style to Sy's guidelines.

After nearly three hours, I learned these ten things about Sy Sperling, enemy of the people extraordinaire:

Sy Is the Spuds MacKenzie of Hair Replacement, a Real Party Animal. When Sy got divorced from his first wife in his mid-twenties, he decided it was time for a change. He reentered the hip singles scene of the 1960s as a hairless guy. But babes weren't flocking to bald Sy. "I'd walk into singles places and I wasn't being responded to the way I'd hoped to be by the other sex. I became socially inactive. When you're twenty-five or twenty-six, it's premature to retire. I liked the idea of [the weave] because you got the results immediately and you could go out that night to a disco and have fun. I didn't go out the first night I had this on, but a week later I went to a singles weekend at Grossinger's. I bought new clothing and got excited about the way I looked.

I saw the way I was getting the responses I wanted. It worked for me."

I guess Sy scored!

Sy's Hair Weave Invention Isn't Really His at All. Sy paid an old Italian inventor in lower Manhattan to train him in a process that weaves pseudo-hair into the side hairs of a baldie. "I was the person who developed it and marketed it and try not to give him credit for it."

Andy Sperling Is Not Only Sy's Son, He's a Client. Andy's twenty-three and, like his daddy, has lost a lot of hair. Just weeks before I met Sy, Sy had a piece made up for his boy. "It's hereditary in our family," says Sy. "The cards were marked." Sy prompts Andy into being a walking familial ad for the Club. Says Andy: "When I used to sleep and touch my head, I'd wonder where my hair was. People looked at me and said, 'You're going bald.' I love this. I don't even know it's there." Sy: "Doesn't he look terrific?" Just like a chip—or strand—off the old block.

Sy Doesn't Keep a Good Secret. During our talk, I mention the newspaper where I once worked. Sy excitedly leaps to his feet and says, "Do you know John ———?" Yes, I do. John is not only a close friend, he's a client! John has appeared in a Hair Club video and Sy obligingly fetches some before-and-after photos of John. It dawns on me that John's pseudo-hair never grew any longer and never budged in the years I knew him. I guess that meant it was reasonably undetectable. But why would Sy reveal this secret about a man with whom I worked? Shame, Sy. Shame. (Sy also tells me about a famous basketball player who is a client, but got fed up with people knowing he was a client, so he asked Sy to stop saying he was a client. So Sy tells me who he is. I won't tell.)

Sy Didn't Always Sell Scalp Covers. No, Sy was not always a hairmeister. He wasn't born the president and a client. He has also sold swimming pools. More important, he has sold—believe it or not—carpeting. When his daughter, Shari, reveals this to me, Sy says, "Oh, don't even mention that. He'll make a joke about it." I'll just leave it where it is, Sy. No jokes. But, Sy, admit it, selling carpets was perfect training.

Sy Doesn't Feel Guilty about Making Bald Guys Feel Guilty about Being Bald. "I don't consciously make bald people feel embarrassed. In my advertising or in the thirty-minute film I'm making, I never once say if you get your hair done here you'll score with women. If you want to stay bald, stay bald. That's fine. I don't criticize that. But if you want to do something, do it. I don't even talk about problems. I say thinning hair, not thinning hair problem. Oh, once in a while a word slips out, but I don't want to offend anyone with thinning hair."

Sy Is Phasing Himself Out of the Hair Club (But He'll Always Be with Us on TV). Now he's only on the haired job three or four days a week, and in a few years, it'll be only two days. He wants to work on charity (free hair for needy bald guys?) and just be a consultant and do grand openings. But thank God, he'll always be the spokesman. He'll never get celebrity fever. "I think there's something very believable about Sy Sperling. He's the guy next door. He has it himself and he talks from the gut. Maybe he has some speech imperfections. But he's real."

Sy's President Once Ran Dunkin Donuts. Yes, it's true. The day-to-day powers in the Hair Club are Sy's wife, Amy, and George Haggerty, the ex–chief executive of Dunkin Donuts. I could swear I almost heard George pacing back and forth in his office, saying dronelike: "Have to make the hairpieces. Have to make the hairpieces . . ."

Sy Wanted to Pick Up Babes When He Was Eleven Years Old. Sy hails from the South Bronx and was first smitten with girls at age eleven. He had hair then, but no moves. So he hung out with Puerto Rican and black guys to learn the secrets of their pick-up lines. "I'll never forget this black guy would go up to a girl and say, 'Hey, mama, what's happenin'. Let's get started.' And she got into his car. I always admired that straightforward philosophy. So after my divorce, when I'd meet a woman, I wouldn't ask her about her birth signs or what college she went to. I'd be more direct. I'd say, 'You're a very attractive woman and I'd like to be with you.' "

Sy Is Taking His Hair on the Road to Moscow. Sy makes his hairpieces in China and Korea, but has plans to build a plant in the Soviet Union to which he'll ship the Indian hair he uses for all the pieces. He'll also open a Hair Club branch in Moscow. "We're doing it for the publicity, not the rubles. We want to show that perestroika starts at the top. We'll try to get Gorbachev to try something on. We want to start it with his hair. It's hairnost!"

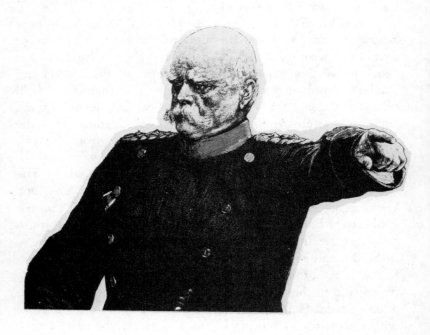

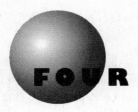

A BALD LOOK AT HISTORY

○

THE UNHAIRED HAVE had great influence on the history of the world, in both good and bad ways. But the history books don't mention the bald view of history, perhaps because the publishing world is dominated by men with too much hair. Nevertheless, after careful research, I, Baldman, have come up with some of the dates the world was inexorably changed by the bald, whether they be great or infamous.

JANUARY

Jan. 1, 1925—Knute Rockne leads Notre Dame over Stanford, 21–10, in Rose Bowl.

Jan. 1, 1975—Watergate baldies John Mitchell and John Ehrlichman are convicted of cover-up charges.

Jan. 5, 1931—Oscar-winning actor Robert Duvall born in San Diego.

Jan. 5, 1964—Led by quarterback John Hadl, the San Diego Chargers win the 1963 AFL Championship.

Jan. 5, 1990—Hockey great Guy Lafleur of the Quebec Nordiques shows off his "hair replacement unit" in *New York Post* advertisement for Manhattan-based hairmeister. According to Lafleur: "People like it. I like it and most of all, my wife likes it. So why not?"

Jan. 7, 1990—All so-called baldness remedies that purport to grow hair—except minoxidil—are banned by the United States Food and Drug Administration on the grounds that they don't do what they promise to do.

Jan. 10, 49 B.C.—Julius Caesar crosses the Rubicon.

Jan. 12, 1971—First episode of *All in the Family*, produced by bald Norman Lear, and costarring prematurely balding Rob Reiner.

Jan. 15, 1967—Max McGee, who didn't expect to play and had caroused the night before, catches seven passes, including two touchdowns, to lead the Green Bay Packers to a 35–10 rout of the Kansas City Chiefs in Super Bowl I.

Jan. 15, 1990—Forty-one-year-old chubby George Foreman continues his comeback by knocking out aging Gerry Cooney in the second round of their fight, dubbed "The Two Geezers at Caesars."

Jan. 20, 1980—Terry Bradshaw leads the Pittsburgh Steelers to a 31–19 win over the Los Angeles Rams in Super Bowl XV.

Jan. 21, 1924—Greatest Soviet pilgarlic, Lenin, dies at age fifty-four, and across the Atlantic, Telly Savalas is born (to be bald).

Jan. 22, 1901—Edward VII, the former Prince of Wales, becomes King of England, succeeding his mom, Queen Victoria.

Jan. 22, 1973—Deliberately shaved head George Foreman knocks out Joe Frazier to win the heavyweight title.

Jan. 23, 1985—Fat chef James Beard dies.

Jan. 29, 1980—Ha-cha-cha-cha: Jimmy Durante dies.

Jan. 30, 1948—Mahatma Gandhi shot and killed by a haired Hindu extremist.

Jan. 30, 1965—Winston Churchill dies.

FEBRUARY

Feb. 3, 1945—Hall of Famer Churchill meets haired FDR and Stalin in Crimea.

Feb. 4, 1969—Bowie Kuhn becomes commissioner of baseball, succeeding bald General William Eckert.

Feb. 5, 1953—Jimmy Durante wins Best Comedian Emmy.

Feb. 6, 1927—Yehudi Menuhin, then seven and hirsute, makes smashing violin debut in Paris.

Feb. 9, 1909—Former Secretary of State Dean Rusk born in Georgia.

Feb. 9, 1914—Maverick baseball team owner Bill Veeck born in Chicago.

Feb. 9, 1955—George Meany becomes head of unified AFL-CIO.

Feb. 10, 1949—Future baldy Arthur Miller's *Death of a Salesman* opens on Broadway.

Feb. 11, 1936—Burt Reynolds born in Waycross, Georgia.

Feb. 11, 1986—Natan Sharansky freed after eight years in Soviet prison.

Feb. 12, 1926—Baseball player–broadcaster Joe Garagiola born in St. Louis.

Feb. 14, 1989—Author Salman Rushdie is sentenced to death by Ayatollah Ruhollah Khomeini because of the allegedly blasphemous offenses against Islam contained in Rushdie's bestselling book, *The Satanic Verses*.

Feb. 17, 1908—The Old Redhead, baseball announcer Red Barber, born in Columbus, Mississippi.

Feb. 20, 1962—John Glenn blasts off in Mercury 6.

Feb. 22, 1918—Ex–baseball team owner Charles O. Finley born.

Feb. 23, 1943—Former Oakland Raiders flanker Fred Biletnikoff born.

Feb. 26, 1973—Noël Coward dies.

Feb. 26, 1979—Evil baldie Khomeini returns to Iran from exile.

Feb. 28, 1916—Snooty novelist Henry James dies.

Feb. 28, 1930—The captain of the Love Boat, Gavin MacLeod, born in Mount Kisco, New York.

Feb. 29, 1952—Dick "Cute as a Bald" Button wins fifth straight men's world figure skating championship.

MARCH

March 2, 1931—Soviet leader Mikhail Gorbachev born.

March 5, 1946—Leave it to a great baldie: Churchill coins the term "Iron Curtain."

March 8, 1973—Watergate baldie Ehrlichman is indicted for his role in the cover-up.

March 11, 1980—Philandering diet doctor Herman Tarnower is put on ultimate diet: lover Jean Harris shoots him dead.

March 12, 1930—Gandhi begins march to Gulf of Bombay and manufactures salt in defiance of British.

March 12, 1966—Bobby Hull, the Chicago Black Hawks' "Golden Jet," breaks his own record of fifty goals in one season by notching his fifty-first.

March 13, 1985—Mikhail Gorbachev, biggest Soviet baldie since Khrushchev, takes over as supreme leader.

March, 15, 49 B.C.—Caesar is stabbed by haired friends.

March 16, 1982—Claus von Bülow convicted of trying to murder his wife, Sunny.

March 17, 1956—Phil Silvers wins Best Comedy Series and Best Comedian Emmies.

March 19, 1985—Joe Pepitone, one of baseball's first toupee wearers, is arrested by police in a car in Brooklyn found to have drugs and a loaded handgun. He would be convicted of misdemeanor drug charges and sentenced to six months in prison.

March 20, 1922—Carl Reiner, a man who knows when to take his toupee off, born in the Bronx.

March 20, 1959—"Hello" Dalai Lama flees Tibet.

March 21, 1927—Chiang Kai-shek takes control of Shanghai.

March 22, 1931—William Shatner born in Montreal.

March 23, 1919—Benito Mussolini forms the Italian Fascist Party.

March 23, 1950—Broderick Crawford wins Academy Award for best actor in *All the King's Men*.

March 29, 1919—Robert Goddard theorizes that man will one day go to the moon, which is shaped like a bald head.

March 29, 1951—His Royal Baldness, Yul Brynner, makes Broadway debut in *The King and I*.

March 29, 1976—Jack Nicholson and his receding hairline win their first Best Actor Oscar for *One Flew Over the Cuckoo's Nest*.

APRIL

April 4, 1954—Arturo Toscanini, at age eighty-seven, conducts for the final time.

April 5, 1945—Churchill surprises everyone by resigning as British prime minister.

April 7, 1920—Indian sitarist Ravi Shankar born.

April 9, 1966—Lucky guy: Carlo Ponti, the Italian film producer, marries Sophia Loren in Hollywood.

April 9, 1984—Duvall wins Oscar for Best Actor for *Tender Mercies*.

April 10, 1949—Slammin' Sammy Snead wins his first Masters by three strokes.

April 11, 1951—General Douglas MacArthur removed from his command in Korea by President Truman.

April 11, 1961—Top bald Nazi Adolf Eichmann goes on trial in a glass booth.

April 13, 1957—With coach Red Auerbach guiding the Boston Celtics' attack and rookie Bill Russell leading the floor attack, the Celtics win their first NBA championship—and the first of nine in a row.

April 15, 1978—*Kojak* airs last episode on CBS.

April 15, 1985—Marvelous Marvin Hagler knocks out Thomas Hearns in the third round of their middleweight title fight, and sets record of fifteen for the most title defenses in his weight class.

April 17, 1966—Auerbach steps down as head coach of the NBA Boston Celtics to become general manager. Bill Russell becomes coach.

April 20, 1986—Vladimir Horowitz returns to Soviet Union for concert after leaving sixty-one years before.

April 22, 1954—Senator Joseph McCarthy starts televised hearings into communism in the Army.

April 23, 1616—Shakespeare dies.

April 23, 1931—Warren Spahn, the winningest left-hander in baseball history, born.

April 25, 1956—Reza Khan crowns himself Shah of Iran.

April 26, 1564—Shakespeare baptized.

April 26, 1984—Count Basie tickles the ivories no more, dies at age eighty.

April 27, 1922—Jack Klugman born, without a toupee, in Philadelphia, Pennsylvania.

April 28, 1937—Heavily receding Jack Nicholson born in Neptune, New Jersey.

April 28, 1945—Benito Mussolini shot dead with his mistress; his bald head later displayed on a rifle butt in Milan.

April 28, 1960—Spahn pitches a 1–0 no-hitter against the San Francisco Giants.

April 30, 1973—Ehrlichman and three haired Nixon aides resign amid allegations of Watergate cover-up.

MAY

May 2, 1903—Baby doctor Benjamin Spock born.

May 3, 1919—Folk singer Pete Seeger born.

May 3, 1976—Sports columnist Red Smith wins Pulitzer Prize.

May 5, 1904—Cy Young pitches the first perfect game of the modern era of baseball.

May 6, 1910—King Edward VII dies in Buckingham Palace.

May 8, 1926—Don Rickles born in New York City.

May 8, 1970—Coach Red Holzman leads the New York Knicks to their first NBA title.

May 9, 1971—Baldies Jack Klugman and Edward Asner take the Emmys for Best Actor in Comedy and Dramatic Series.

May 10, 1940—Churchill takes over as British prime minister, vows "nothing to offer but blood, toil, tears and sweat." He can't offer his hair.

May 10, 1973—Holzman leads his New York Knicks to their second NBA championship in four years.

May 13, 1981—Pope John Paul II is wounded by a haired Turkish assassin outside Saint Peter's in Vatican City.

May 17, 1976—Asner wins Emmy for Best Actor in a Drama, *Rich Man, Poor Man*, proving the versatility of bald actors.

May 18, 1930—Pernell Roberts born, without his toupee, in Waycross, Georgia.

May 18, 1937—Hall of Fame third baseman Brooks Robinson born.

May 18, 1977—Menachem Begin leads Likud Party in elections and becomes Israeli prime minister.

May 19, 1974—French go for it: elect bald Valéry Giscard d'Estaing as president, succeeding bald Georges Pompidou, who succeeded bald Charles de Gaulle.

May 20, 1927—Soon-to-be-bald Charles Lindbergh leaves Long Island for history-making flight to Paris.

May 20, 1981—Another hairless French leader, François Mitterand, is elected president.

May 22, 1962—E. G. Marshall wins Emmy as Best Actor for *The Defenders*.

May 22, 1966—Sam Denoff and Bill Persky win Emmy Award for Best Comedy Writing for episode of *The Dick Van Dyke Show* in which Laura Petrie (Mary Tyler Moore) reveals to the world that Alan Brady (Carl Reiner) is bald.

May 23, 1945—Churchill resigns as prime minister and calls for new elections.

May 23, 1960—Israelis capture Eichmann.

May 27, 1936—Louis Gossett, Jr., born in Brooklyn.

May 28, 1974—Patron saint Savalas wins Best Actor Emmy for the first season of *Kojak*.

May 30, 1908—Mel Blanc, the voice of Bugs Bunny and Porky Pig, is born.

May 30, 1961—A. J. Foyt wins his first Indianapolis 500 title, completing 200 laps in 3 hours, 35 minutes, 37.49 seconds.

JUNE

June 1, 1909—W. E. B. DuBois forms the National Negro Committee.

June 3, 1921—Beat poet Allen Ginsberg born in Paterson, New Jersey.

June 4, 1987—Hurdler Edwin Moses's streak of 122 consecutive victories in the 400 meter hurdles is broken in Madrid.

June 5, 1963—Who says bald men aren't sexy? Bald British pol John Profumo resigns after charges he had sex with prostitute Christine Keeler.

June 5, 1982—Thoroughbred trainer Woody Stephens wins first of five Belmont Stakes races as Conquistador Cielo wins with Laffit Pincay aboard.

June 6, 1944—Hall of Famer Dwight Eisenhower leads Allied troops on D-Day invasion.

June 9, 1914—Senator Alan Cranston born in Palo Alto, California.

June 11, 1990—Joe Garagiola returns as cohost of the *Today Show*, proving NBC found that only a great bald man could save the morning program.

June 12, 1901—French physicist Henri Becquerel discovers radium.

June 13, 1989—Kareem Abdul-Jabbar plays his final game in pro basketball as his Los Angeles Lakers lose the NBA championship series to the Detroit Pistons. The forty-two-year-old Abdul-Jabbar ends his career as the game's greatest scorer.

June 15, 1752—Ben Franklin flies a kite, proves lightning is electricity, makes few remaining hairs stand on end.

June 15, 1976—Joe Frazier comes out completely bald during his second bout with George Foreman. This might have been a precursor for Foreman eventually shearing his hair.

June 17, 1966—Rubin "Hurricane" Carter is arrested for the murder of three in a New Jersey barroom—charges that he would fight for two decades before his eventual release.

June 18, 1976—Toupee wearer Charles O. Finley's attempt to sell three of his top Oakland A's is voided by Commissioner Kuhn.

June 25, 1982—George Shultz replaces combover wearer Al Haig as secretary of state.

June 29, 1956—Arthur Miller proves bald men are sexier by marrying Marilyn Monroe in London.

JULY

July 2, 1881—James Garfield becomes second president to be assassinated.

July 3, 1957—Khrushchev foils a coup against him.

July 4, 1826—John Adams, second bald president, dies (on same day as haired president Thomas Jefferson).

July 4, 1910—Heavyweight champion Jack Johnson knocks out Jim Jeffries in Reno, sparking riots.

July 9, 1968—Harmon Killebrew ruptures himself on a long stretch at first base during baseball's All-Star Game.

July 11, 1920—Soon-to-be-national holiday: birthday of Yul Brynner, in Sakhalin, Japan.

July 11, 1969—Baby doctor Benjamin Spock's conviction on conspiracy to counsel draft evasion is overturned by an appeals court.

July 12, 1952—Eisenhower nominated in Chicago by Republicans to run for president.

July 14, 1913—Gerald Ford born in Omaha, Nebraska.

July 14, 1967—Milwaukee Brave Eddie Mathews hits his five hundredth home run.

July 16, 1948—Leo Durocher quits as manager of the Brooklyn Dodgers to run the New York Giants.

July 18, 1921—Former astronaut Senator John Glenn born in Cambridge, Ohio.

July 22, 1959—Khrushchev and Nixon engage in Kitchen Debate in Moscow, set up by semibaldie William Safire.

July 23, 1945—One bald Brit, Clement Attlee, replaces another, Churchill, as British prime minister.

July 25, 1959—Khrushchev and Nixon debate further in Moscow kitchen.

July 26, 1926—William Jennings Bryan dies, five days after winning conviction of John Scopes in Monkey Trial in Tennessee.

July 26, 1952—Military officers in Egypt oust King Farouk and replace him with his son.

July 26, 1952—Adlai Stevenson named by Democrats to face Ike in presidential election.

July 27, 1906—Leo Durocher born.

July 28, 1978—Another Rickles show, *C.P.O. Sharkey*, bites the TV dust.

July 31, 1983—Brooks Robinson, enemy of the people in his toupee, is inducted into the baseball Hall of Fame.

AUGUST

Aug. 1, 1956—Jonas Salk's polio vaccine made available to the public.

Aug. 9, 1974—Bald vice-president Gerald R. Ford becomes first bald (if unelected) president since Eisenhower.

Aug. 9, 1988—Upjohn gets approval to sell baldness "cure," minoxidil, to the public.

Aug. 10, 1948—Allen Funt, TV's chief voyeur into the lives of Americans, debuts *Candid Camera* on ABC.

Aug. 12, 1984—Killebrew, who hit more home runs than any other bald man, is inducted into the baseball Hall of Fame.

Aug. 20, 1951—Hockey legend and future hairpiece wearer Guy Lafleur born.

Aug. 21, 1965—Astronaut Pete Conrad blasts off in Gemini 5 with haired Gordon Cooper for 120 orbits of Earth.

Aug. 25, 1920—Sean Connery born in Edinburgh, Scotland.

Aug. 31, 1958—Olympic hurdler Edwin Moses born.

SEPTEMBER

Sept. 2, 1948—Former quarterback Terry Bradshaw born.

Sept. 2, 1966—Hiding beneath his toupee, William Shatner starts life as Captain Kirk on *Star Trek*.

Sept. 4, 1957— Baldman born.

Sept. 5, 1927—Former Federal Reserve Board chairman Paul Volcker, the man who saved America's economy, born in Cape May, New Jersey.

Sept. 5, 1929—Button-down and balding Bob Newhart born in Oak Park, Illinois.

Sept. 6, 1901—William McKinley is second bald president assassinated.

Sept. 7, 1963—Warren Spahn wins twenty games for the thirteenth season.

Sept. 7, 1988—Drexel Burnham junk bond king and bad toupee owner Mike Milken is indicted.

Sept. 8, 1974—President Ford pardons Nixon.

Sept. 8, 1977—Zero Mostel dies.

Sept. 10, 1973—As a bus company lost and found custodian, Dom DeLuise debuts in the sitcom *Lotsa Luck.*

Sept. 10, 1986—Laurence Tisch succeeds in ousting CBS's overhaired chief executive officer, Thomas Wyman, and takes over the entertainment conglomerate.

Sept. 11, 1924—Football coaching legend Tom Landry born.

Sept. 12, 1977—Louis Gossett, Jr., wins Emmy for Best Actor in a Dramatic Series for his role as Fiddler in *Roots.*

Sept. 12, 1989—Ed Koch loses his bid for a fourth term as New York City mayor when David Dinkins defeats him in the Democratic primary.

Sept. 15, 1938—Spitball pitcher Gaylord Perry born, gurgles up first ball of saliva.

Sept. 15, 1940—Texas chrome dome Sam Rayburn elected speaker of the House of Representatives—the first of his three tenures as head of the House.

Sept. 15, 1960—Warren Spahn pitches a 4–0 no-hitter against the Philadelphia Phillies.

Sept. 16, 1914—Allen Funt, creator of *Candid Camera*, is born.

Sept. 17, 1900—William Jennings Bryan accepts the Democratic nomination for president.

Sept. 17, 1968—Gaylord Perry of the San Francisco Giants pitches a 1–0 no-hitter against the St. Louis Cardinals.

Sept. 17, 1978—A Baldie Bonanza at Emmy Awards: honors to go to Ed Asner, Michael Moriarty, Rob Reiner and Tim Conway.

Sept. 20, 1917—Boston Celtics president Red Auerbach is born in Brooklyn.

Sept. 22, 1902—Actor-director-producer John Houseman born.

Sept. 23, 1952—Eisenhower calls Nixon "my boy," vindicating Nixon in his slush fund scandal, which Nixon explained away in the legendary Checkers speech.

Sept. 23, 1987—Director-choreographer Bob Fosse dies.

Sept. 24, 1955—Leo Durocher zips his lip, quits as manager of the New York Giants.

OCTOBER

Oct. 5, 1947—Red Barber makes classic call of Brooklyn Dodger Al Gionfriddo's catch of Joe DiMaggio's 415-foot drive to left field that subdued the Yankees: "Gionfriddo's back, back, back. Ohhhhh, doctor!"

Oct. 6, 1908—Wilbur Wright sets new record by flying for an hour with a passenger in his flying machine in Kitty Hawk, North Carolina.

Oct. 6, 1981—Bald Egyptian leader Anwar Sadat assassinated.

Oct. 6, 1989—Dalai Lama awarded Nobel Peace Prize.

Oct. 10, 1935—Bald spot owner George Gershwin sees his opera, *Porgy and Bess*, open.

Oct. 10, 1985—Patron Saint Yul Brynner dies.

Oct. 12, 1960—Angered by a speech by a Filipino delegate, Khrushchev bangs his shoe on a desk during proceedings of the United Nations.

Oct. 13, 1970—Dazzling fielding plays and a two-run double by Baltimore Orioles' Brooks Robinson lead his team to a 2–1 lead in the World Series against the Cincinnati Reds.

Oct. 14, 1947—Chuck Yeager breaks the sound barrier in a Bell X-1 rocket plane.

Oct. 14, 1976—Yankees first baseman Chris Chambliss hits the dramatic game-winning ninth-inning home run that beats the Kansas City Royals in the American League playoffs.

Oct. 16, 1981—Greatest bald, one-eyed Israeli, Moshe Dayan, dies.

Oct. 17, 1978—Karol Wojtyla is elected Pope John Paul II.

Oct. 20, 1925—Art Buchwald born in Mount Vernon, New York.

Oct. 21, 1958—After Gracie Allen's retirement, toupee wearer George Burns launches a new sitcom; it lasts one season.

Oct. 24, 1926—Former Giants and 49ers quarterback Y. A. Tittle born.

Oct. 24, 1973—Telly Savalas debuts as the first sexy, lollypop-sucking bald detective, Kojak.

Oct. 26, 1951—What an incredible bald guy: Churchill returns for a second time as British prime minister.

Oct. 28, 1962—Perfect baldie Khrushchev backs down from Kennedy in Cuban missile crisis.

Oct. 30, 1922—Mussolini invades Rome, staging his bloodless coup.

Oct. 31, 1938—John Houseman helps Orson Welles scare the nation with radio broadcast of *War of the Worlds.*

NOVEMBER

Nov. 5, 1952—Greatest election in Bald Presidential History: Eisenhower defeats Stevenson.

Nov. 6, 1956—Second-greatest election in Bald Presidential History: Ike beats Stevenson again. Never again will two baldies face off against each other in the big contest.

Nov. 7, 1917—Lenin leads Bolsheviks to overthrow Russian government.

Nov. 9, 1952—Israel's first president, Chaim Weizmann, dies.

Nov. 13, 1964—St. Louis Hawk Bob Pettit becomes first National Basketball Association player to score 20,000 points.

Nov. 14, 1900—Composer Aaron Copland born.

Nov. 15, 1929—Ed Asner born.

Nov. 20, 1910—Leo Tolstoy, still sporting a long compensatory beard, dies.

Nov. 20, 1977—Anwar Sadat addresses Israeli Knesset.

Nov. 20, 1987—Don Zimmer, known affectionately as either "Popeye" or "Gerbil," is named manager of the Chicago Cubs, having already managed the Boston Red Sox, Texas Rangers and San Diego Padres.

Nov. 22, 1963—Semibald Lee Harvey Oswald assassinates John F. Kennedy.

Nov. 23, 1929—French premier Georges Clemenceau, who negotiated the World War I treaty in Versailles, dies.

Nov. 30, 1916—Austrian emperor Franz Joseph dies after sixty-eight years on his throne, the longest reign of any bald monarch.

DECEMBER

Dec. 1, 1935—Woody Allen born in Brooklyn.

Dec. 2, 1942—Physicist Enrico Fermi and his team in the Manhattan Project create the first nuclear reactor.

Dec. 2, 1954—Hall of Shamer Joe McCarthy is censured by the Senate.

Dec. 5, 1935—Humorist Calvin Trillin born in Kansas City.

Dec. 6, 1968—General William Eckert is fired as commissioner of baseball.

Dec. 10, 1907—Rudyard Kipling wins Nobel Prize for Literature.

Dec. 10, 1976—Economist Milton Friedman wins Nobel Prize.

Dec. 10, 1978—Begin and Sadat win Nobel Peace Prize.

Dec. 12, 1905—Pavlovian response: Ivan Pavlov wins the Nobel Prize for his dogs, who salivate on command.

Dec. 12, 1915—The Chairman of the Board of Hairpieces, Frank Sinatra, born in Hoboken, New Jersey.

Dec. 12, 1932—Bob Pettit, the first superstar basketball forward of the 1950s, is born.

Dec. 12, 1964—Y. A. Tittle plays his last game—the "Bald Eagle" retires number 14.

Dec. 12, 1977—New York's bald demigod, Ed Koch, is sworn in as mayor of the city for the first time, on his fifty-third birthday.

Dec. 13, 1920—Former Secretary of State George Shultz, the most ovoid bald head since old Citizen Kane, born in New York.

Dec. 13, 1981—Sharpshooting NBA guard Lloyd B. Free of the Golden State Warriors changes his first name to World, and subsequently says he might name his son Second World and Third World.

Dec. 15, 1933—Tim Conway born in Willoughby, Ohio.

Dec. 17, 1903—Balding Wright brothers take flight for first time in their airplane at Kitty Hawk.

Dec. 19, 1960—Charles O. Finley buys a controlling interest in the Kansas City Athletics; a few years later, he'd ship them off to Oakland.

Dec. 21, 1975—Denver Broncos running back Floyd Little retires.

Dec. 22, 1968—David Eisenhower, bald like Grandpa Ike, marries Julie Nixon.

Dec. 23, 1948—Tojo, Japanese military leader in World War II, is hanged with six others.

Dec. 24, 1943—Ike takes over the European Front for the Allies.

Dec. 29, 1982—Alabama football coach Bear Bryant retires.

Dec. 31, 1943—Actor Ben Kingsley, who would win an Oscar for playing the bald Gandhi, born in Yorkshire, England.

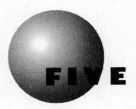

FIVE

BALDNESS IN SPORTS, OR, "HOLY COW, HE'S OUT . . . AND HE'S BALD!"

O

WHEN SPORTSCASTERS SPOT a bald athlete, they react as if they'd found he had no penis. Patron Saint Joe Garagiola recalls hearing an announcer say, "Here comes the reply, watch this play, watch it, watch his hat . . . Denny Walling is bald!" Isn't that special?

Baldman admits that unhaired athletes are an unusual sight. Athletes in their twenties and thirties are less likely to be bald than competitors on golf's Seniors Tour (though old golfers still keep their hair too long; thank God for Tom Weiskopf and Sam Snead, but why isn't Steve Pate bald?). They are young, strong, muscular, square-jawed and haired. Groupies follow them in haired heat; it's rare to see panting women proposition a squad of bald men (a circumstance that would be the girls' loss, not the guys'). Hair remains, to my chagrin, a sign of youth and dynamism; without it, goes the putative mythology, you're as useless as a hairless Samson.

Athletic prowess often equals hair—except if you're a swimmer who shaves his head to pick up speed or Edwin Moses, who lost his protein naturally and went on to Olympic hurdling glory. Think of the greatest athletes of their days: Joe DiMaggio and Joe Namath. Arnold Palmer and Wayne Gretzky. Bjorn Borg and Eric Heiden. Orel Hershiser and Muhammad Ali. All are haired icons. Johnson's Baby Shampoo (which pays Hershiser to endorse its product) would no more approach George Foreman to be its spokesman than Brylcream would come to Ray Nitschke. (Although for guys like Ray, a little dab would have done them fine for a long, long time.)

The youth of athletes usually means a scarcity of baldplayers, and the scant supply is *very* noticeable. And on the field of play, everybody notices it. Thus, even Baldman is surprised when a pilgarlic pro passes before him.

New York has been blessed with two distinguished basebaldies with the Mets and Yankees. Sometime Mets catcher Barry Lyons—successor to overhaired Gary Carter—has taken a lot of clubhouse ribbing, but his scalp has kept on ticking. He's walked around the dugout capless, covering up only on the field. I'm told he's sensitive about it, but he hasn't let it show. Baldman nearly cried when overhaired Mets management sent Barry to the minors during the 1990 season—for one obvious reason: He didn't have enough hair to truly succeed Gary Carter. Shine on, Barry. And Baldman worries about Yankees designated hitter—first baseman Steve Balboni. Steve's pate is as painfully shy as the rest of him.

Baldman weeps for Balboni as he does for ex–Phillies and Reds catcher Andy Seminick. As one story goes, Andy once faded back for a foul pop and knocked his cap off. So embarrassed was Andy at showing his bald head that he covered his scalp with his mitt and let the ball fall.

Sighting baldplayers is a hobby of mine.

During the 1989 World Series, the San Francisco Giants' hard-hitting third baseman Matt Williams, only twenty-three, frequently lost his cap to proudly show a widening crown of hairlessness. He's well on his way to becoming the Y. A. Tittle of baseball.

Then there was New Orleans Saints rookie quarterback John Fourcade removing his helmet on a Monday night football telecast to show a perfect bald spot! I got three rapid-fire calls from my crack crew of bald-spotters on this sighting. And up in the announcing booth that day, a rearview shot of Frank Gifford and Al Michaels revealed two fine domes in the making.

Baldman sees pilgarlics everywhere—and eagerly seeks them out when he can. Imagine the glee of sitting down to breakfast at an All-Star weekend in Cincinnati with a venerable quartet of ovoid legends—Leo Durocher, Enos Slaughter, Luke Appling and Warren Spahn. Scalp Heaven!

For many Bald-Stars, hairlessness came late in a career or in retirement. Some lose it naturally; some shave it off. Kareem Abdul-Jabbar did both. Think of Kareem through his career and you'll remember two extremes: in his UCLA and Milwaukee Bucks years, he had a large Afro, but as the years went by with the Los Angeles Lakers, his hair started disappearing until he had a bald spot that seemed to grow by the minute. Finally, Kareem shaved it all off—and now it's easier than ever to spot him in a haired room.

Baldplayer stories frequently emerge from false hair. One of the classics is Joe Pepitone, the mischievous ex-Yankee, known during his career for introducing the hair dryer to the clubhouse—but more important, for his collection of hairpieces. Joe wore one during the game and another for his varied social life.

Hockey superstar Bobby Hull is one of the first known players to have gotten a transplant. I'm sure Bobby's hair loss was painful psychologically, especially because his nickname was "The Golden Jet." The transplant never took well. These days, Bobby's brother, Dennis, a fine bald left-winger himself, has been heard to joke: "There is one toupee in the family and tonight it's Bobby's" and "Bobby's had more wives than he has hairs."

Hull has a soulmate in another hockey great, Guy Lafleur. In his 1988–1989 comeback year with the New York Rangers, Lafleur was bald. When he moved to the Quebec Nordiques for the 1989–1990 season, I got a call from Paul, my hockey-writer friend, to report the appearance of an unidentified haired object perched on Guy's head. As if to confirm it, Guy soon appeared in a hairmeister ad, which said: "Lafleur is one of the few players in hockey who still plays without a helmet. More startling, he wears a hair replacement unit both on the street and on the ice. Perhaps most remarkable of all, it stays put. Always. Without exception." With enough glue, anything can stay on, Guy.

I'd prefer that Lafleur and Hull follow the lead of Ivan "Ching" Johnson, a New York hockey great of the 1930s, who sported a full head of skin and no regrets. One account described him as a "bald and amiable" defenseman who'd slam you into the boards with "impartial cheerfulness."

Speaking of cheerfulness, who could be a cheerier baldie than George Foreman? When he was haired, he was a nasty, dour monster who followed the personal lead of the felonious Sonny Liston. In retirement, he found God, flab and a shaved head. Not surprisingly, in his comeback, he's a happy man, refusing to say a bad thing about his opponents, but still pummeling them with his fists. He may look like a forty-two-year-old Buddha, but he's content. The hair was evil. Being bald has made the difference for his psyche and his aerodynamics.

There are other stories of bald redemption. Through his career, Pittsburgh Steelers quarterback Terry Bradshaw lost his hair and started wearing a hairpiece that formed only a light patina of protein over his tundra. But in recent years, as his broadcasting career took off, off came his rug—and danged if he didn't look as good as ever.

There are also stories of false-haired bravado occasioned by the wearing of evil false hair by the moguls of sport. Take Charles Finley, who was awfully proud of his hairpieces. Writer Murray Chass recalls approaching Finley in a Philadelphia coffee shop to talk to the former Oakland Athletics owner.

"He was showing off the piece," says Chass, "and at one point, he's talking about how he attracts young girls when he's wearing it. He said, 'Look at that table, they can't take their eyes off me.' I said, 'Charley, one of those girls is my wife, and she's just waiting to see me stop talking to you."

The first superstar baldplayer I noticed growing up in the 1960s was Green Bay Packers linebacker Ray Nitschke, old number 66, the man who revolutionized his position in the pre–Butkus and Lawrence Taylor days. Ray was a ferocious player who lost his hair in his early twenties and never paid it any mind. In an exclusive talk with Baldman, he said: "I never even thought about it. I just accepted it. It was never that important. My father had a good head of hair, but I lost mine. I took some abuse for it, but it wasn't that bad. It didn't bother me. Nobody got on me too much."

Did the smooth exterior enhance his ferocity? "I don't know, but it was very noticeable. It became a trademark. I feel like I never age."

Ray was once a guest on the *Today Show*, with Garagiola. During a commercial break, they both put on hairpieces. Ray recalled: "I felt different. I felt like a different person when I had hair. I wasn't my normal self. I talked and acted differently. I wasn't the same character when I was bald."

Ray's wife, Jackie, one of nature's noblewomen, met her future husband when he had lost nearly all he had! "He thought he had a crewcut, but he was bald. It never bothered me, and I came from a family with a lot of hair. I don't think about people's hair. That time he tried on the hairpiece, he came home with it, and it looked real terrible."

The Nitschkes—a couple bound in beauteous baldness.

Baldman sees hope on the horizon, in the soaring, flying body of Michael Jordan, the Chicago Bulls' superstar guard. One NBA executive said I should place Michael on the basketball bald-star team because of his shaved head, which he says was occasioned by a rapidly receding hairline. I examined Michael's head, and I see a hairline of stubble. Maybe Michael knows more about his hairline than I can determine on television—and maybe he is going bald naturally. Whatever the reason, I think it's fair to say that Jordan is the Telly Savalas of sports: a man at the top of his game who sees value in being clean-shaven. So Michael, for as long as you keep the hair away, long may the wind blow through your follicles as you climb ladders of air to slam dunk —and may the scalp be with you.

BALDMAN'S ALL-TIME BALD-STARS

In creating Baldman's All-Time Bald-Stars, I tried to be as complete as possible, but I'm sure I missed some fine unhaired stars. It was tough to find photos of unadorned players who wear caps or helmets but I reveled in creating the basketball list for they all play in their underwear. I also discovered that football garb provides an interesting twist: in their helmets, all players are bald.

```
    *    reputed toupee wearer
   **    reputed hairweaver
  ***    reputed minoxidilist
 ****    shaved head
```

BASEBALL
p: Warren Spahn, Nolan Ryan, Gaylord Perry, Rick Reuschel, Cy Young, Phil Niekro,* Luis Tiant
c: Gene Tenace, Joe Garagiola, Barry Lyons, Haywood Sullivan, Andy Seminick*
1b: Harmon Killebrew, Vic Power, Chris Chambliss

2b: Johnny Temple* Art Howe
ss: Cal Ripken, Jr., Dick Groat, Spike Owen
3b: Brooks Robinson,* Eddie Mathews, Sal Bando,
Howard Johnson, Matt Williams
of: Reggie Jackson, Ken Singleton,** Enos Slaughter, Joe
Pepitone,* Denny Walling, Ruppert Jones, Ron
Blomberg, Joel Youngblood***
dh: Steve Balboni
manager: Leo Durocher
coaches: Roger Craig, Rube Walker, Walter Alston,
Joe Altobelli, Art Howe, Lee Walls****

BASKETBALL
centers: Kareem Abdul-Jabbar,**** Nate Thurmond,
Zelmo Beatty
forwards: Bob Pettit, George Yardley, Rick Barry,**
Toby Kimball, Granville Waiters
guards: Michael Jordan,**** Slick Watts,**** Xavier
McDaniel,**** Gus Williams, World B. Free, Bobby
Weiss, Curly Neal,**** Red Klotz
coaches: Jack Ramsey, Red Holzman, Alex Hannum
gm: Red Auerbach

FOOTBALL
Offense
qb: Y. A. Tittle, John Hadl, Terry Bradshaw
rb: Floyd Little, Rocky Bleier, John Riggins****
recs: Joe Morrison, Fred Biletnikoff, Max McGee,
Carroll Dale
line: Bob Keuchenberg, Ray Wietecha, Mike Webster,
Henry Jordan, Jack Stroud, Lenny St. James, Fuzzy
Thurston, Reggie McKenzie, Joe DeLamielleure
k: Garo Yepremian, Don Chandler
p: Dave Jennings

Defense
line: Bob Gain, Willie Davis, Otis Sistrunk,**** Floyd
Peters, Ernie Holmes****
lb: Ray Nitschke, Dan Curry, Jack Pardee
db: Mel Renfro, Herb Adderley, Neil Craig, Dick
Pesonen, Mel Blount, Mark Murphy
head coach: George Halas

HOCKEY

goalies: Billy Smith,* Roger Crozier
centers: Doug Mohns,* Lorne Henning,
Bobby Sheehan, Howie Morenz, Jacques Lemaire,
Donnie Marshall
wings: Bobby Hull,*,** Guy LaFleur,* Ross Lonsberry,*
Dennis Hull, Dave Ballone, Wayne Cashman
defense: Ivan "Ching" Johnson, Jack Crawford, Bill
White, Gary Bergman
head coach: Billy Rey

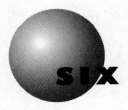

LOOK, UP IN THE SKY, IT'S A BIRD! IT'S A PLANE! NO, IT'S A BALD ASTRONAUT!

○

WHEN HE WAS asked the traits for a perfect astronaut, veteran haired Soviet cosmonaut Yuri Romanenko, who at the time had spent more than ten months in space, suggested that he or she should have:

- Huge arms—six preferably.
- Slim legs—one skinny limb would be best.

And, most important:

- A bald head—to avoid haircuts.

Hair flopping around in space would seem to be a nuisance. Baldness would seem to improve an astronaut's aerodynamics—especially in space walks.

I believe that the high point of the United States' space program was the flight of Apollo 12 when two bald astronauts, Charles Conrad and Alan Bean, walked on the moon, leaving behind their haired colleague, Richard Gordon, to do the boring stuff up in the air. The previous flight, Apollo 11, featured balding Buzz Aldrin walking on the moon—but he did his walking second, behind haired Neil Armstrong, a clear case of anti-baldness prejudice. But lest we forget, the first astronaut to orbit the Earth, John Glenn, was bald. They used a haired guinea pig—Alan Shepard—to get into space, but when it came to a really important mission, they went to a baldie!

So NASA deserves a Bald Man Government Service Award for its role in making baldies a priority in space. Helmets off to the great baldonauts of NASA:

    First Team: John Glenn
                  Charles Conrad
                  Edwin "Buzz" Aldrin
  Second Team: Michael Collins
                  Alan Bean
                  Tom Stafford
   Third Team: Ronald Evans
                  Tom Mattingly
                  Charles Fullerton
  Fourth Team: William Thornton
                  Alfred Worden
                  Rep. Jake Garn

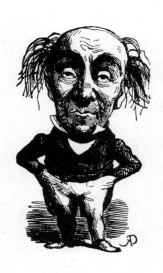

RICH MEN, BALD MEN

Money is a democratic commodity: whether it is earned, saved or spent, it doesn't ask how much hair you have. The success of all but one of these ten billionaires (save for Michael Milken, who allegedly wears an obvious toupee) shows that hair might have blocked their view in pursuit of bald wealth.

1. John Werner Kluge, Metromedia—$5.2 billion*
2. Ted Arison, Carnival Cruise Lines—$2.86 billion
3. Ronald Perelman, Revlon—$2.75 billion
4. Henry Lea Hillman, industrialist—$1.7 billion
5. Samuel LeFrak, real-estate developer—$1.7 billion
6. Forrest Mars, Sr., Mars candy empire—$1.5 billion
7. Walter Annenberg, publishing—$1.4 billion
8. Laurence Tisch, CBS and Loews—$1.35 billion
9. Ewing Kauffman, Marion Laboratories—$1.3 billion
10. Michael Milken, ex–Drexel Burnham Lambert financier—$1.27 billion

Source: *Forbes* magazine (1989).
*At about $1,200 per hairpiece, Kluge could buy 4,333,333 rugs, or 26,000 Hair Club for Men franchises, at $200,000 apiece.

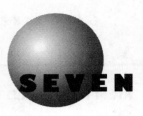

SEVEN

AND NOW ... THE PATRON
SAINTS OF BALDNESS!

○

JOE GARAGIOLA

OH, GOD, WHAT PURPOSE HAS BEEN SERVED?

Name: Joe Garagiola
Occupation: Cohost, the *Today Show*
Started Balding: Late twenties
Minoxidil Opinion: Wouldn't try it
Toupee Opinion: Okay for others, not him
Time for Haircut: Twenty minutes

BALDMAN: When you get up in the morning and look in the mirror, what do you see?

GARAGIOLA: I don't see myself as bald. I've looked at myself for so long. Carl Reiner's my hero. He goes on the *Tonight Show*, he puts on his toupee one time, another time he doesn't. It's just the way he wants to dress tonight. Like I want to wear this tie tonight, but I won't wear it tomorrow night.

B: When did you start losing it?

G: I was in my late twenties. A baldheaded guy never thinks he's going bald. You're just losing a little bit of hair. And all of a sudden, you realize, "Oh, oh, what's happening here? There's more in my comb than there is on my head."

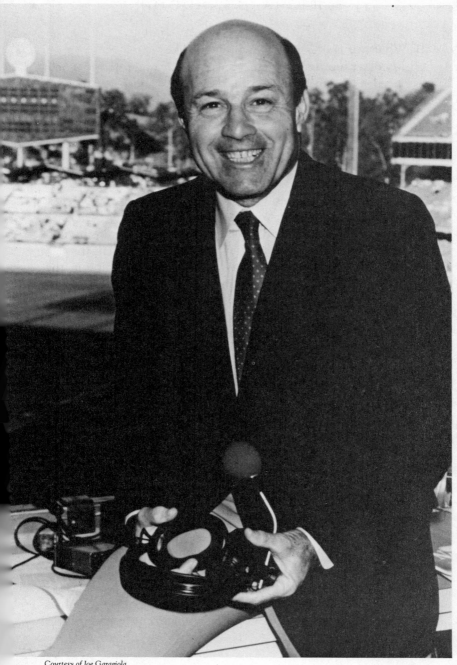

Courtesy of Joe Garagiola

B: What was the Garagiola family hair like?

G: My older brother can get a crewcut today and tomorrow he'll need a haircut. He's got a widow's peak and he's two years older than I am. Very little gray. I mean healthy hair. My father had plenty of hair. My uncle was bald. My mother had plenty of hair.

B: How about your mother's father?

G: I didn't know any of my grandparents because they were all over in Italy. I don't remember seeing any bald family pictures until I started appearing in them.

B: Were you this bald in your twenties?

G: I wasn't that bald when I was playing. But I was losing it. I was in the shock stage, the trauma stage. Then I went through the stage when I figured this wasn't the worst thing in the world that could happen to me.

B: Ballplayers can be vicious. Did they rag you?

G: Every line referring to it was a cutting line. People start talking to your hairline instead of into your eyes. Once it's gone, ballplayers jump all over it. I used to get Dick Groat real bad at home plate. I started discussions about going bald with him during the National Anthem and he hated it. A lot of baldheaded guys won't come out for the National Anthem. You know, most catchers are bald. But are they catchers because they're bald or bald because they're catchers?

B: Did they call you any particularly nasty names?

G: I'd get called chrome dome and skinhead. "Keep your hat on the glare's killing me," they'd say. My hero as a ballplayer was Andy Seminick, who was bald and was the only guy who could slide and if his hat came off, he would catch it and put it right on. I thought he had the hat tacked on because it hardly ever came off. Howard Pollett was my roommate and he was bald, so we had no problems.

B: Who was the first toupee wearer you knew of?

G: Tony Lupien. He was with the White Sox. Joe Pepitone had a gamer toupee and one for after the game. He had a little blowout patch for his bald spot. A little Saint Anthony's patch.

B: You've made good fun of yourself, but were you always so well adjusted to being bald?

G: You think, "Why me, why me, oh, God, why me?" You look at some guy, like a priest at Mass, with a full head of hair, and you say, "What does he need it for?" That's just the beginning when you lose your hair. I think you come to where you accept it and there's not a darned thing you can do about it. When I was doing the *Today Show*, it got to be like Dear Abby. I'd get letters from young women who'd write to me and say, "We're going to get married in three months and my boyfriend is so worried that he's losing his hair and I always point to you and say, 'Look, he's not worried and I love you for what you are. I don't care if you're bald.' " I'd have to sit down and write letters to these guys and I did. It may be funny to some people, but to a person who's undecided about what to do, it's really traumatic.

B: When did you accept it?

G: I'll tell you when. I was in the last stage, where I had that one healthy strand on the wrong side of my head, and I'd go across with it. And I was doing the Bob Hope Desert Classic with Bob Prince and Jim Simpson and Lindsey Nelson. And they all had their hair. Lindsey has a high forehead but plenty of hair. Well, they took a high shot of us when they taped the opening. I had combed the strand straight across and from the high shot, I couldn't believe what I looked like. It looked like Highway 66 running across my head, like some giant varicose vein. And I looked at that and said, "Oh man." I was in my late thirties or early forties.

So I was doing the *Today Show* and I just told the gal to snip the strand right off. I thought, "What am I going to do, get a toupee? Or go like this?" I just watched other guys with toupees and it just wasn't me and I said, "Well, this is it. That's the way the Lord wants me."

B: Did you ever wear a toupee?

G: I put one on during the *Today Show* and people really wrote in. It was the day General Gavin was on and he gave his platform for running for president. Hardly any reaction to him. But the toupee? We were flooded with mail. Put it on. Don't put it on. We got everything.

B: Ever think of using minoxidil?

G: Not at my age. But I'll tell you what. One of my fantasies is on a TV show to be miked and have cameras hidden, put on a toupee and walk into a clubhouse just to see what the guys would say. It would be hilarious. I have a toupee at home. My wife once suggested I dress up for dinner at home, and put the toupee on. The dog started barking like crazy. He didn't recognize me.

B: Transplants?

G: I remember when people like Hugh Downs and William Proxmire got transplants. I saw those plugs, man. They were ugly. Looked like someone ran over their head with track shoes.

B: What do you do about haircuts now?

G: I pay full price. But see, I'm a tough haircut. Billy Consolo, who was a ballplayer, was also a barber, and I said one day, "How would you cut my hair?" He said, "You're a tough haircut. You got a bunch of guys waiting, so I gotta make it last twenty minutes. You know how hard that is?"

B: Did you ever suffer antibaldness discrimination?

G: We *are* discriminated against. It was hinted to me to think about putting on a toupee at NBC. But nobody really asked me. I was going into sports and baldness was more accepted. I'm a pioneer because I was the first bald game show host and with the *Today Show*, I broke the ice. But you hear, if I'm standing next to someone who has to be pointed out, "He's standing next to the bald guy." You don't hear, "He's standing next to the hairy guy."

B: What's the absolutely worst thing you've ever seen happen in baseball to a bald guy?

G: How about this? I'm watching TV and Denny Walling of the Astros made a diving catch and his hat came off and the announcer said, "Here comes the replay, watch this play, watch it, watch his hat," and he says, "Denny Walling is bald!" And I said, "I can't believe he said that." The next night, Buddy Bell made a similar play and his hat came off. I called the announcer and said, "Why didn't you say Buddy Bell is hairy?"

B: Do you feel a special kinship with bald guys?

G: When two baldheaded guys talk, it's like the Born Again movement. We're born again bald. We accept it. Accept it? You have no choice, although the choice may be a toupee. I have yet to see a guy wearing a toupee who can get by a plate glass window or a mirror without checking to see if it is still on. My wife and I can spot a toupee blocks away. I've seen some bad ones, boy. I mean, some come from the looms of Mohawk. Different colors, some that look like they were thrown up, and some guys are buying it by the pound! One week you'll see it and it looks okay, and the next week you say, "Whoa, what growth!" So I'll tell my wife, "That's a rug." It's like a game. The only guy I ever said anything to was this guy who'd put me down. He was drinking too much. When I got alone with him, I said, "Let me tell you something. I'm blowing your cover. If you think you're fooling me with that rug you've got on, you're crazy." And he got all shook up. But we baldheaded guys become experts on this. That's one thing we notice.

B: Ever wish for hair now?

G: As a believer, I think that maybe when we get to the Big Bullpen in the Sky, we'll have five questions to ask. And one of the questions I'm going to ask is, "Why do I have so much hair on my chest and so little on my head? What purpose has been served?"

SENATOR ALAN SIMPSON

BALD GUYS—LIKE GORBACHEV AND HIM—ALWAYS GET THINGS DONE

Name: Alan Simpson
Occupation: United States senator from Wyoming
Started Balding: Early thirties
Minoxidil Opinion: Wouldn't try it
Toupee Opinion: Okay for others, not him
Transplant Opinion: Must be painful

BALDMAN: You are certainly, in my mind, the leading bald senator, but then there aren't too many of you. Is it tough to be bald and in national politics?

SIMPSON: I can't believe that. I know there are photogenic men with dazzling heads of hair. But I just never think of that. It's funny. When I see someone with a hairpiece, I kind of shudder. I've never seen one that really looks good. I'm sure there are some that are very expensive and dazzling. One time I put one on and wore it for a half a day, and people looked at me, thinking, "I wonder, did he have cancer? Does he have pernicious anemia?" It was the damnedest thing.

B: Did you wear it in the Senate?

S: No, no way.

B: Did you ever feel yourself succumbing to the transplant option, like former Senator Proxmire did?

S: I've never felt that need. I know others want to. If they want to, that's fine, I guess, but I can't imagine having a grain drill going through my head.

B: Did you ever get up close to Proxmire's head? What did you think of it?

S: All I can say is it must be painful. That's my first thought. It's something people want to do. Strom Thurmond did it. If they want it, more power to them.

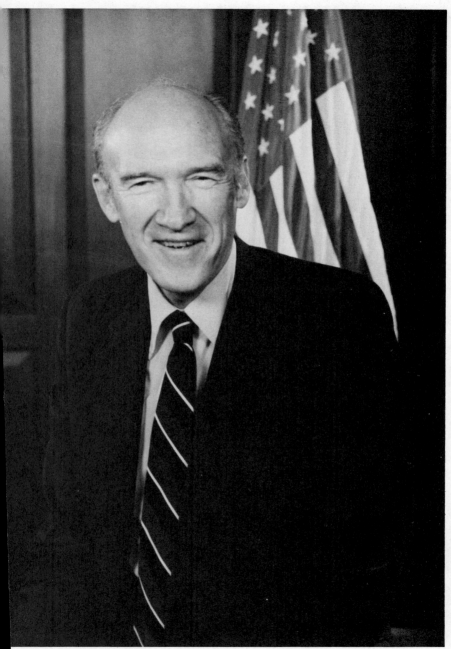

Courtesy of Senator Alan Simpson

B: What do you think of Senator William Roth's hairpiece?

S: I didn't know for a while that he had one. I didn't know until I saw a picture of him in his home. I saw a photo of this good-looking bald guy and I said, "Bill, who is that handsome guy, your brother?" He said, "No, it's me." I don't think people immediately recognize it as a hairpiece. He's very well groomed.

B: Do you think there will ever again be a bald president? Baldness and the White House just seem mutually exclusive.

S: I don't think it has anything to do with it. It used to be that hair and religion meant something, but they're pretty well gone now. I don't think of it as a hindrance at all. I've never felt any limitation in my life, in any form, from being bald.

B: It would seem for us baldies that our favorite elections were the 1952 and 1956 Eisenhower-Stevenson elections.

S: Well, I never thought of them as my favorite elections because they were bald. But Ike was attractive, which kind of puts the lie to the notion that a bald guy can't look good and be president. Stevenson looked good, too. I just suppose it is less likely to be a bald president because there are fewer bald men than men with hair. So therefore, fewer run for president.

B: Have you ever talked to Senators Alan Cranston and John Glenn about being bald?

S: Al and I kid each other. People come up to me and call me Cranston. I say to Al, "Do people call you Simpson?" He said no. How come they call me Cranston?

B: Maybe they can't tell us bald folks apart.

S: Maybe. People also confuse me with Senator Leahy. We both have glasses and whitish hair. The odd thing is they confuse me with other guys but never do they get asked, "Hey, are you Alan Simpson?"

B: Maybe you're not as well known or as powerful as I thought you were.

S: When you're a Republican from a state of 460,000, you don't think of yourself as well known.

B: When did you start balding?

S: Honestly, I don't know. I'd have to look back at pictures of myself, because I never thought of myself as losing hair. I guess I was in my thirties.

B: You're known as a funny guy willing to poke fun at your baldness. What are some of your jokes?

S: There was one attributed to me that wasn't mine. This bald guy in Cheyenne came up to me, said "Aha, Simpson," and patted my head. Well, I started to pat his head, and he said, "Don't touch me, it's a solar panel for a sex machine." Then Jake Garn talked about not wasting your hormones on growing hair. You always get a lot of mileage by making fun of yourself. I was out getting a hunting license in Wyoming and the lady clerk there nailed me on catastrophic health care. So she's talking and I say, "But could you get me my license?" She said, "I'm not through with you." So, in the blank on the license that asks about hair color, she wrote "glossy."

B: Can you think of any bad things that have happened because you're bald?

S: Oh, people kid you. They call me chrome dome and those things. That's part of life. I'm a great kidder. I like it. I've never felt offended by people calling me chrome dome.

B: Some people think that the combination of your height and baldness give you a very powerful look.

S: I don't think of myself as powerful. I've never felt that. You feel power in your heart, I guess. I'm self-conscious about being tall. I slump a lot. Sometimes, I shlump around so that I can hear people. What being tall does is make you very noticeable. I walk down the street in Washington or Cody, Wyoming, and people recognize me. I'm very tall and very bald so my visage is something you remember.

B: Did your wife ever mind that you are bald?

S: She never said a word. I married a classy chick thirty-five years ago. When I got married I had a full head of hair. My nickname was T.C., for Tony Curtis. It was naturally curly and there was so much of it. Then it just slowly disappeared. I don't remember it going down the drain or falling out on my pillow. As my wife, Anne, says, "You're more attractive now than when we were married." My sons, I can see that they're losing a little. They know what's ahead of them.

B: So you've never been denied a job, a promotion or housing because you're bald?

S: No, I never, never, never felt discriminated against by being bald. People gravitate toward you. They say, "Hey, baldie." A guy who's bald and truly enjoys it is a gregarious kind of guy, a salesman. They tell great stories. It's tough to generalize so much about a group, but bald guys who have confidence in themselves have an extra edge. They learn to handle things.

B: If you had to give advice to a bald guy who couldn't accept his hair loss, what would it be?

S: That's tough. I'm sure it must be tough for some people. I'd tell them to quit watching those stupid ads on television, where my God, they make you call a number, and you think it's to call a doctor to check on this supposedly grievous situation and it's for a medicated product that they're selling. It's so phony. I think you just have to be who you are. Self-esteem is the most important thing in life. I'm not talking about arrogance but I'm talking about self-esteem. It's taking the package God gave you. I have a nose that looks all mashed down; it looks like a ski slope. I have a physique like a crane. But I like myself. Unless you like yourself, you have a lot of problems. If you compare yourself to other people, the very act of comparing me to anyone automatically puts me in second place and second place is a poor place to start. Instead of comparing, just say, "I'm bald as a billiard ball." Think of Yul Brynner and the powerful sex symbols of the past. The great genies of the Arabian Nights. What's that they say? "For all sad words of tongue and pen. The saddest are these: 'It might have been!' "

B: Do you attach much significance to the fact that the bald Mikhail Gorbachev is the first Soviet leader in a while to be making forward progress?

S: I just don't think it has to do with him being bald. I know he wears a hat like I do. If I didn't wear a hat, I'd perish.

B: But you have to admit that this bald leader is finally getting things done in the Soviet Union.

S: Bald guys always get things done. They are a spirited bunch and they really seem to be an extra special, virile, exciting group to be around.

B: Are you rooting for his survival because he's bald?

S: No, I root for him so mankind can succeed.

B: Senator Simpson, you are a great bald man.

S: Thank you, and good luck to you.

JERRY DELLA FEMINA

DON'T MESS WITH HIS SHAVED HEAD

Name: Jerry Della Femina
Occupation: Chairman of Della Femina, McNamee WCRS, New York advertising agency
Started Balding: Twenty-two to twenty-three
Minoxidil Opinion: Wouldn't try it
Toupee Opinion: Like false teeth
Time for Haircut: Who needs a haircut? He uses an electric razor.

BALDMAN: I notice from some photos that you once had hair around the edges.

DELLA FEMINA: Now I shave it every day.

B: With what?

DF: A regular shaver. I do it by sound. I can hear the crackling sound. When the sound ends, I'm done. I enjoy doing it. I've done it for seventeen years.

B: Ever cut yourself shaving?

DF: It's an occupational hazard. When I'm away on vacation, I go two or three days without shaving. It starts to come in and boy, do I move fast to shave it. I don't like the sense that there's any hair.

B: What made you do it?

DF: I hated being bald. I really truly hated the concept of balding. It's a lifetime sentence. There was no way out of it. You could buy a hairpiece but you'd look like a fool. The concept of a hairpiece is disastrous. It's like false teeth. It's sad. At the same time, it would be nice to have hair. So I found myself between two things.

B: How did you go out and do it? It's not an easy thing to do.

DF: One day I said I had to do something. I didn't want to wear

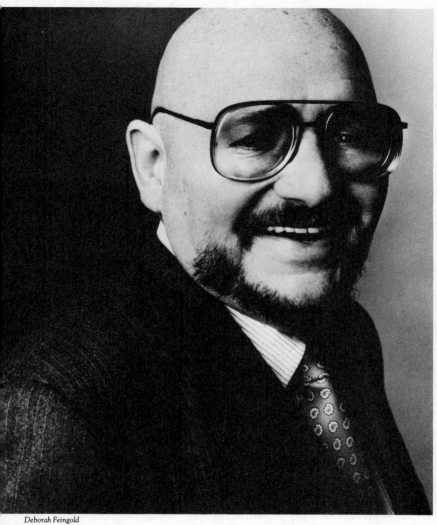

Deborah Feingold

a hairpiece. So I went to Gio, my hairstylist. Before I left, I told my three-year-old daughter, Jody, "I'm going to come back without my hair." And she was all psyched up that daddy was going to come home different. So I went to Gio and he charged me twenty-five dollars to shave off the fringe.

B: Twenty-five dollars just to shave off the sides?

DF: Yeah. He must have said, "This man is a fool, but I'll never see him again. This is the last twenty-five dollars I'll ever make from him." So he shaved it off. I know I could have done it myself, but I didn't think I could bring myself to do it. Who knew what was under there?

B: What was the reaction?

DF: I came home, opened the door and Jody started screaming and crying. Then I did something really wise. I opened my head out of town. Just as you do it with shows out of town. I went to Palm Beach. I did it for two reasons. I think a bald man with a tan looks better. So I got a tan. And I wanted to get used to myself when people were talking to me, to get a sense of how they felt. I was out of town for ten days and by the time I came back, people were running up to me, rubbing my head. That was fine. In a month, nobody paid any attention.

B: Any other changed attitudes?

DF: People got a totally different view of me. They thought I was tougher and meaner. I'm not tough and mean.

B: Now you're a buccaneer.

DF: The view was, "I don't want to mess with this guy." Same guy. Just a few hairs gone. Before that I was a sedate pussycat. Same people. It shows what hair means.

B: I know tanning my bald head is an invitation to pain and peeling. What's your tanning secret?

DF: My skin. I have real Mediterranean olive skin. I just sit out there in the sun.

B: No sun block.

DF: No. No sun block.

B: So now you have a look.

DF: Oh, yeah. Women say that. I was on a plane. A woman sitting across the aisle keeps staring at me. She was well-dressed. In first class. She came over and said, "Can I touch your head?" I said, "Sure." She said, "I was just imagining what it felt like." It's a head. My head. I suppose it looks better than it feels. It's just an expanse of hard skin with no stubble on top.

B: How did being bald make you feel?

DF: Bad. Nobody said anything to make me feel that way. At that point, they can't make you feel any worse than you feel for not having hair. So I found myself becoming more socially aggressive. I'd say being bald had a real effect on my personality. You compensate.

B: How does being fully shaved feel?

DF: I love it. Now I'm not bald anymore. I don't see myself as a bald man at all. Not in the slightest.

B: What is your label then?

DF: I'm a man with a shaved head. My face has become ageless. People tell me the same thing. I looked older twenty years ago than I do now. It drove me crazy that when I was thirty-three I looked forty-three or fifty-three. Shaving it takes the age out of it. The image is younger.

B: Doesn't your head get cold in the winter?

DF: I don't wear hats. I don't like the look of a hat without hair. It's ridiculous. I just felt if I didn't have hair, I'd get rid of everything.

B: A shaved head distinguishes you.

DF: I feel like I did something definite, that I really dealt with being bald. In a sense, I have more control over baldness than I ever did. You control it or it controls you. It's great. It's me. If someone came out with a pill that would give me a full head of curly hair tomorrow, I wouldn't take it because I'm so happy shaving it all off. My wife can find me in any restaurant. I'd never want to have hair.

B: Ever wear a hairpiece?

DF: Years ago, my first client was a hairpiece manufacturer. Squire for Men.

B: What a beautiful irony.

DF: The first ad they did won every big award. The headline was "Are You Still Combing Your Memories?" I wrote it. It's the best piece of copy I ever wrote. I wrote another headline that said, "I Hate Being Bald." The client insisted that I put a hairpiece on. He was crazed that I wouldn't up until then. But it was good. He took a Polaroid of me. I brought it home to my first wife. I woke her up and said, "Look at this. Do you recognize this person?" She said, "This is someone we both know but I can't figure out the name." That's how different I looked. I looked good, but it struck such a false note.

B: How old were you when you lost your hair?

DF: Twenty-two or twenty-three.

B: What was your reaction?

DF: Horror. It was very traumatic, especially in my twenties. The people around me didn't mind.

B: They never tell the truth.

DF: Yeah, families do that.

B: Was there a lot of baldness in the family?

DF: I understand one's mother's brother is a good gauge.

B: How bald was your uncle then?

DF: Bald, of course. He combed it way over, trying to get the most of his seven or eight strands.

B: How's your older son's hair?

DF: Good. He's got a full head.

B: What do you think of minoxidil?

DF: When it came out, people said, "Why don't you use it?" Why? Why should I go back and look like everybody else when I can be a part of what is a fairly striking minority?

B: We bald folk are a second-class minority, aren't we?

DF: It's a respect thing. Bald people don't get the same respect.

People with full heads of hair are treated one way. People with little hair are treated another way.

B: Your profession, advertising, has done a lot to foster the view that hair is virility, that hair is power.

DF: Sure. You don't see many bald models, unless you specifically need one. The father in commercials isn't balding. I think advertising contributes to the idea that you're not as good as anybody else, that you're not in the mainstream.

B: Do you work against that by going out of your way to cast bald models?

DF: Not really. Even when I was balding, I'd say, "Why cast a bald model?"

B: Shame on you.

DF: There just aren't that many of them. I think it would be more natural if commercials showed more bald guys. It would be closer to reality. It goes to the myth that a bald guy can't sell things as well. Ever see a bald guy in beer commercials? Does a bald guy stand around and say, "Here's to good friends and Löwenbräu"? Out of six guys, shouldn't one of them be bald? In real life, one of them would be.

B: Have you ever been denied a job or promotions because you were bald?

DF: No! What I have felt is when I go into a room where a CEO is bald, I feel a kinship. I feel we share something. Not that we exchange a secret handshake, but I feel he's more comfortable with me.

B: Feel more sympathy for a bald job applicant?

DF: No. On the contrary. I think I treat them the same way other people treat them. I perpetuate the feeling.

B: Hmm, this is disturbing. I don't know if you can continue as a Patron Saint.

DF: I'm being truthful. I don't treat them the way they should be treated. I guess we turn on our own.

B: Don't you think guys with bad combovers should just shave them off and be aggressively bald?

DF: I think everybody should shave it off. That's the answer.

B: Do you need the right shaped head for a shaved look?

DF: I don't know. Everybody I've seen with their head shaved looks fine. Once you know it's gone, it's pretty neat. You ever toy with shaving it off?

B: Me? No. I haven't had the nerve.

DF: We'd probably look like doubles if you did.

DICK VITALE

I'M A BALD, ONE-EYED WACKO!

Name: Dick Vitale
Occupation: College basketball commentator on ESPN and
  ABC-TV
Started Balding: Early twenties
Minoxidil Opinion: Not a chance, baby
Toupee Opinion: No way
Time for Haircut: Five minutes

BALDMAN: When did you lose your hair?
VITALE: Very young. When I was in my early twenties. It was
  all shedding little by little. When I got involved in coaching,
  I had a big crop of hair. Then they told me that I had to
  win all the time and I lost it all. By thirty, I was bald big
  time, baby. But I was sexy. People ask me, "Dick, how did
  you get such a gorgeous wife?" Bald is beautiful, baby, bald
  is sexy. No rugs get on my scalp. It's what I am. I'm a bald,
  one-eyed wacko.
B: How old were you when you met your wife?
V: Twenty-nine.
B: So you were totally bald at that time. What did she say to
  you when you started dating?
V: She said she never thought she'd marry a guy who was bald
  or heavy. That really turned her off. But she just looked
  deeper into the person. I tried to woo her with my personality
  and charm, because I couldn't do it with my hair.
B: Did it bother you to lose your hair so young?
V: I never felt any form of depression or any vanity about it. No
  down moments because I was losing my hair. It was just a
  part of life. I've seen so many successful bald people in sports
  that I felt being bald was a break. What bothered me more
  was my eye. I lost it and it drifts. That's what my parents

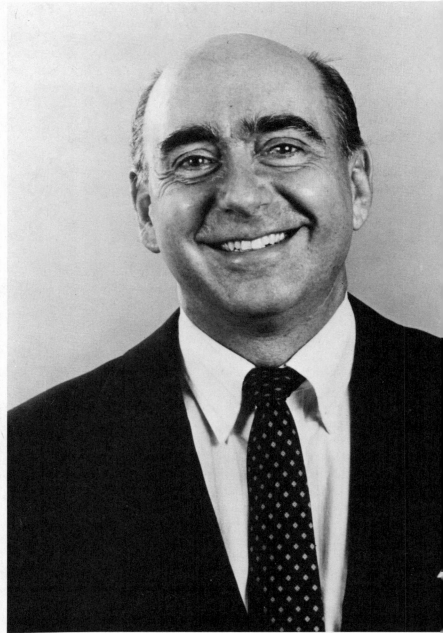

were more worried about. But never the loss of hair. Maybe my up-tempo personality compensated for it.

B: Your parents must have instilled a lot of confidence in you that made you have that attitude.

V: I had tremendous love at home. My parents had a fifth-grade education but a doctorate in love. The guidance they gave me really helped.

B: What's the baldness situation in your family?

V: My father is bald. He's lost a lot of hair. My brother has a thick crop.

B: Are you jealous of him?

V: No. Never. Sometimes, I'll be at banquets and I'll see people with lots of hair and I'll kid 'em, "With your hair, I could be a big TV star."

B: You are, of course, a TV star, and being bald must create some occupational hazards.

V: Oh, yeah, I drive people in TV crazy because the lights beam off my dome. Drives 'em nuts! But it's a way of life. You can't hide from that.

B: Did ESPN or ABC ever say, "Dick, it might be a good idea if you had some hair"?

V: Not to my knowledge. I've been on ESPN for eleven years and they just signed me to a five-year extension.

B: How has the haired world mocked you?

V: Oh, I really get it at Duke. When I walk out, half the crowd starts chanting, "Bald." The other half chants, "Head." Then together they chant, "Bald Head. Bald Head. Bald Head." I drive 'em crazy. I take out a comb and I make like I'm combing a few strands. The place goes bananas. They yell at me. "Hey baldie!" I never take it too seriously. I have too many things to worry about. Too many of us look in vain for things like this. It's nice to look good. We all want it. But there are more and better things to be occupied with.

B: They must get on you at other colleges.

V: The Duke and Syracuse fans really yell at me. They do it lots of places. Especially if I say something that's not positive about their team. So the quickest thing is for them to yell out, "Hey baldie!" It's like the baldness is supposed to rattle you. It just makes me smile. I take out my comb and it drives them totally bananas.

B: The locker room is usually a pretty ribald place. How did your players get on you for being bald?

V: Sometimes guys shine your dome and joke around. But you laugh about it. People get on people if they know they're sensitive about a particular thing. But I just laugh.

B: In the pro coaching world, where you spent some time, the greatest coaches have been bald.

V: Right. Auerbach. Ramsey.

B: Holzman.

V: Right.

B: You see any connection between baldness and great coaching?

V: I never think of a coach being great because he's bald. I don't look at people that way, as being bald or having a thick crop of hair. I feel you judge a person as what they are as a human being, not whether they're short or tall, fat or thin.

B: What does it say about a country that is so hair-crazy?

V: There are other things to worry about than losing hair. There are lots of good-looking people who are bald. The worst thing is when you see guys with toupees who cover their baldness and baby, they just look way out! It stands out so badly.

B: Ever tempted to wear one?

V: Only on Halloween. I figure it might really be a shock. My next thing is to show up for a game wearing a thick crop of hair. It would probably ruin my image. I'm a baldheaded guy.

B: Do you think hair transplant places should be banned?

V: (Laughs.) I know a bald guy who had a transplant. Very successful guy. He said he'd spent over twenty-five thousand dollars to have it done. He said he went berserk watching his hair fall out. He couldn't stand to see it. I said, "You can't be serious, worrying all the time about your hair falling out." I can see worrying if it was a disease. But never. I'd never do anything like that.

B: I hate the ads where they say, "Cure baldness."

V: Yeah. Like it's some disease.

B: Would you ban any hair replacement establishments?

V: Well, I don't know why anybody would want to go through that cycle. But to each their own. It's their bodies. I guess they'd have to shut down all the toupee places if everybody had my attitude, baby.

B: Ever think of shaving it all off?

V: No. It always drove me nuts watching people take a few strands and comb it over the top. I did that when I was in my late twenties. But there were strands all over the place. It was so uncomfortable. I used Vitalis to keep it down. I still use Vitalis every morning, but I don't think I'd be a good walking advertisement for them. You know, nobody ever said I was on TV because I looked like Robert Redford.

B: Ever been denied housing or a job because you were bald?

V: No, but I guess I was denied a few dances when I was younger.

B: How do you think you look bald?

V: I look younger now. I stopped wearing glasses. I'm not heavy. I looked older when I was younger. Now I look young for my age.

B: What's the absolute worst thing that ever happened to you because you're bald?

V: The only bad thing is how quickly I'm out of the chair for a haircut. I pay $6.50 or $7.50 and I'm out in five minutes.

MIKE ROYKO

WOMEN WHO HATE BALDIES ARE NINNIES

Name: Mike Royko
Occupation: Syndicated columnist, the *Chicago Tribune*
Started Balding: Forties
Minoxidil Opinion: Wouldn't try it
Toupee Opinion: Won't wear one
Time for Haircut: Fifteen minutes

BALDMAN: When did you go bald?

ROYKO: I'm fifty-seven now, and I started losing it when I was about forty.

B: Is being bald something you've thought much about?

R: It wasn't unexpected because my father lost his hair at about the same age, and it was the same pattern. I have a brother who's two or three years older who looks like he's wearing a monster hairpiece, except it's his own hair. So I knew that I'd probably lose mine. When it started happening, I didn't mind the hairline receding, but when I started getting a bald spot, and it thinned on top, I was self-conscious. But I'm not anymore. By the time I was in my late forties, the deed had been done. I just stopped thinking about it. When I did think about it, I thought about the advantages, especially when I'd finish playing handball and my younger opponents, having lost to me, would be spending all this time with hair dryers in front of the mirror. One of them is a TV reporter, and I'd see how much time he'd spend drying. By the time he'd be finished, I'd have showered, shaved and was just about gone. I figured if he did that every day, he'd be wasting a year of his life blowing hot air onto his head. That was reassuring.

B: As one of the country's foremost big-city columnists, you have

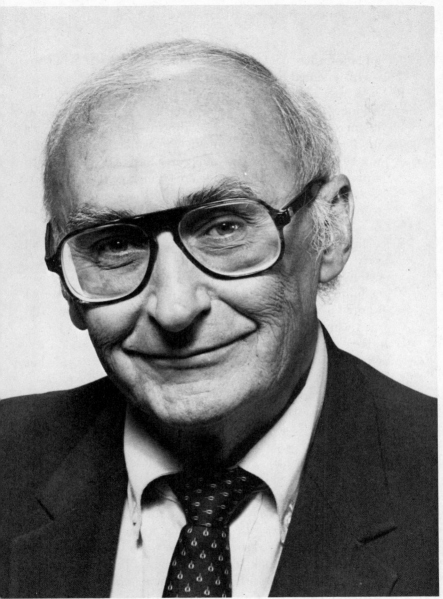

a platform few bald men have. Have you written about the slights endured by many bald men?

R: I've written about it because people will make comments about baldness, not to me, but in general. I've written about how it's an excellent barometer of the intelligence or lack of intelligence of people. A man who winds up marrying a woman who finds baldness important has spent his life with a ninny. Whereas more intelligent women have no interest.

B: You got a lot of negative comments from women in response to your column on *People* magazine's selection of Sean Connery as *People* magazine's 1989's Sexiest Man Alive.

R: I'd say those women are stupid or malicious. They were all very angry at me, because I mentioned cellulite. ["May the cellulite be with you," he wrote.] They have no control over cellulite, but they could go out and exercise their asses. I wanted to zap them where they hurt, because there are bald men who are sensitive.

B: In your commentary on the Connery selection, you said you were pleased and amazed. I understand being pleased, but why amazed? Just that you never thought a bald guy could get that honor?

R: I was lying. I was amazed, but then I thought about how smart *People* was. *People* would not get a syndicated column out of me if they'd named Tom Cruise or any other movie star. It was very shrewd. So I said amazed because Connery is a guy older than me and bald. I wouldn't have been amazed if Yul Brynner were named the sexiest man alive. I saw him in his last road tour for *The King and I*, and the highlight was when he took his curtain call. He still maintained the royal pose and we were his royal subjects. Here was a bald guy looking like we all could look. Part of Connery's thing is that he's in good physical shape, he looks menacing, and he's got good features. The same thing could have been said about Yul Brynner.

B: Was there only that overwhelmingly negative response by women to Connery?

R: Afterward, I received an extraordinary number of letters, from women of all ages, who thought it was a great idea. One woman in her twenties said he has "something" and that baldness was irrelevant.

B: So while we praise Connery, do we also wish that mean old men with lots of hair would finally go bald?

R: No, I just give my brother the needle. He looks more like my son. He looks a lot younger, period. Jim Hoge, the publisher of the *Daily News*, and I aren't far apart in age and we both started as young reporters and we went to a lot of parties together. Then we stopped talking for a couple of years. When he became editor of the *Sun-Times* and *Daily News*, we had a drink together. He said, "Why did we stop being friends?" I said, "It's your fault. You didn't have the decency to develop wrinkles, get fat or go bald. If you lost a little hair, I'd have felt a little bit better." I admit that I was a little envious of him, but it's the Dorian Gray thing. There's probably a picture of him in his attic where he looks like a wreck.

B: Have you ever done silly things, to cover up your baldness?

R: You're the first person I admitted this to: it was eighteen years ago, and it had become acceptable to wear a hairpiece. A number of guys at the *Chicago Daily News* wore pieces, and I wondered what it would look like, so I went over to this hairpiece joint and the guy said, "You really haven't lost that much." I said, "Well, that's the idea." A lot of guys who wear hairpieces, they get them that start around their eyebrows. Bing Crosby, John Wayne and the guys in the old movies had slightly receding hairlines. Sinatra. So if you wear one, it shouldn't look like a Bushman or Lon Chaney in *The Wolf Man*. So I got one. I went on vacation in Florida for two or three weeks, and people said the tan made me

look great, and no one, including my own children, knew I
had the damned thing on. My brother didn't know.

B: So it was a natural-looking one.

R: It had the same hairline I had. It was the same shade of hair.
So I'd been wearing it about two or three weeks and I was
playing handball with my closest friend. We got tangled up
on a shot and I got in his way and he swiped at the ball and
hit my head, and he jumped back with this shriek of horror
because the hairpiece came down over one of my eyes. The
tape had come loose and he thought he'd crushed my head.
He was howling and then he looked at me and said, "Are
you wearing a goddamned wig?"

B: Double-backed tape tends to lose its stickiness in extreme cold
and when you're sweating.

R: Well, that was the end of it for me. I said this is it.

B: How much had you paid for it?

R: About $250.

B: Do you notice the second-class treatment bald men get?

R: I haven't seen much of it. People don't say anything to me
because I have a reputation for being mean. I hear more
ridicule directed at guys wearing hairpieces. A guy I worked
with at the *Daily News* was prematurely bald. He was a
bachelor and well-liked by everyone at the paper. But he
was accident-prone. He wore the piece for two days and
stopped. I said, "Ed, if you're going to wear it, wear it." He
said that wasn't it, but he had left it out one night and the
cat played with it and tangled it up in knots. Then, later,
he went on a date with a woman he'd just met, and the next
day, he said he had a terrible experience. They were sitting
there and she looked at him strangely. He excused himself
to go to the men's room because he thought he had something
on his face. But when he had taken his hat off in the restaurant, some of the tape got loose and his hair was off to
one side. Then one day, it blew off right in front of the
paper. He was chasing it down the street in the middle of

winter. He was chasing his hat as it blew into the river and the hairpiece as it blew down the street. A bus driver stopped, and everybody on the bus cheered. He still wears it.

B: With the legendary winds in Chicago whipping hair about, is Chicago a good place to be bald?

R: Chicago is not as cosmetic, not as fashionable as New York, and it's not as appearance conscious as L.A. One's bod isn't an obsession as it is in L.A. My guess is that hairpieces per capita would probably be lower in Chicago, Pittsburgh and Milwaukee than San Francisco, L.A. and New York. Not that we're square, but we're not that concerned with style. A guy working to make a buck won't worry about spending time every day taping or tacking the hairpiece. Another guy at the paper looked just like Phil Silvers, and he got one. He was in his fifties, and I'm not clear why he did it. One day he sat near me and he was wearing a Cubs cap. I said, "Where's your piece?" He said, "It's in the cleaners." I said, "You have to have two so you can wear one while the other's at the cleaners." He wanted a hairpiece but he was too cheap to buy two, so every few weeks, for a day or two at a time, he'd work with a Cubs cap on.

B: I'd imagine that anyone who wants to test the wind resistance of a hairpiece should come to Chicago.

R: Yeah, I guess. There's a guy named Paul Fenimore in Chicago who's got Hair Line Creations and they did a lot of TV advertising. He hired athletes—not the stars, but middle-level guys—and would show them, like a Cubs third baseman, without his hairpiece. He was really an ugly bald guy. No question. Then he showed him with a Hair Line creation, and he was just an ugly guy with hair.

B: What do you think of hair replacement?

R: If it makes you feel better, it's okay.

B: But guys like us can spot hairpieces a mile away.

R: I can't. Not the real good ones. There's a guy at my golf club who started wearing one. He's thinning but not totally bald.

When he mentioned that he wore one, I was surprised. I didn't know. In his case, he didn't wait until he was totally bald, which is the smart thing to do. I can see someone in the entertainment field doing it. Frank Sinatra probably looks better with a modest piece. Bing Crosby probably prolonged his career because of one. People equate it with youth and vigor. I remember an editor who was in his fifties, a very youthful guy, and he was an editor when I got my column. I remember when I saw a picture of him, I said, "Wow, he was bald. I hadn't noticed." He'd kept his hair fairly short, so you didn't notice his baldness because his hair was just short in general. I went to the barber shop, about a year and a half ago, and I said, "I want it short, as short as a crew cut plus a quarter of an inch." She couldn't believe it. But when she finished, she said, "Now I see what you mean, you look much younger." Now I do it often. It's my Mussolini look. I pay eight bucks for about fifteen minutes.

B: Were you ever interested in taking minoxidil treatments?

R: No. If there were something with a 50 percent success rate with guys who are really bald, I'd blow the dough. Apparently, there's only limited success with minoxidil—those who are very young and who are starting to get thin. A TV guy I worked with at the *Sun-Times* has had transplants and they seem to have worked. He's in TV, but without too many exceptions, people in TV have hair. If I were in a field where the roof over my head depended on my having hair, I'd do what had to be done.

B: What did your wife think when you lost your hair?

R: Oh, she didn't care. She was one of the intelligent ones. You know, there are some funny things guys do to hide baldness. Some guys use a dark spray on a bald spot. I knew a circulation guy at the paper and we were sitting together, and I looked at his head and said, "For Pete's sake, Joe, you're spraying your head." He said, "You shouldn't have noticed." I said, "You're short, if you were taller I wouldn't have noticed."

I once called up tattoo parlors to see if they tattooed hair on heads. Some guys had tattooed hair. It was effective if you were two blocks away. We had a bald guy in Chicago who was about six-foot-six, and eccentric. He'd gone to a tattoo parlor and you'd see him on the Loop. When he bowed, you'd see the top of his head. On top, there was Jesus' face.

B: Do you suspect that journalism treats its bald better than other image-conscious professions like entertainment?

R: Yeah. By the time you get into the world of grown-ups, the amount of hair you have shouldn't be a factor. Surely at the top levels. Both guys who run this company are bald.

B: Did you ever feel prejudice because you were bald?

R: No. You have to remember, I started my column when I was thirty-one, and won the Pulitzer Prize when I was thirty-nine, and I had a book, *Boss*, that was a big best-seller before I was forty. So I had pretty much made it in my chosen work when I still had my hair.

BERNIE SIEGEL, M.D.

IF YOU HAVE SELF-ESTEEM, DON'T CARE IF YOU HAVE NO HAIR

Name: Bernie Siegel
Occupation: Surgeon, now self-healing guru, author of the best-selling book *Peace, Love and Healing*
Started Balding: Early twenties
Minoxidil Opinion: No need for it
Toupee Opinion: Ditto
Time for Haircut: As long as it takes to lather up and shave

BALDMAN: I'd known about you for a while, but when I saw that beautiful picture of you and your bare head on the cover of *New York* magazine, I knew you had to be a Patron Saint.

SIEGEL: Well, thanks.

B: So when did you start losing your hair?

S: Somewhere back in my college days. In my twenties it began to go. And it was never anything that I had any thought of trying to reverse or stop or change or have surgery for. At that time, our generation wasn't into those things. It never was a question to me that there was anything to do about it. It was perfectly natural.

B: But some people have always wanted to cover up.

S: Sure there were some people. But I don't like anything artificial. I just wanted to be me. My father was bald and it wasn't any big deal.

B: What did your family and friends say?

S: I can't remember anybody saying anything about it. It was never an issue.

B: Did it hurt your social life?

S: No. I was married at age twenty. By the time I was a med student, I was married. So there was no effect.

B: What was losing your hair like?

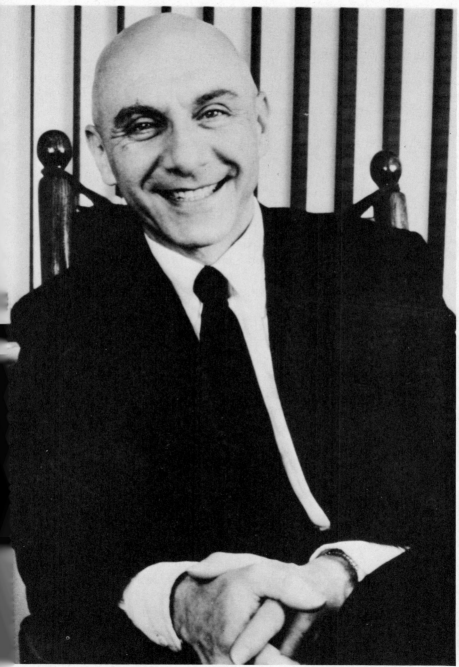

Thomas Victor

S: A nuisance. But I saw people growing it long to comb it over, then it went up in the wind. I just made it short. It was a lot easier that way. As a child, I had nice wavy hair. It went from one end of the spectrum to the other.

B: Eventually, you shaved all your hair off. Why?

S: I'd had a great urge to shave it for several years. This urge goes back twelve or more years when I finally did it. When I did it, some people were angry at me for being different. They'd stop and yell at me. Somebody I met yesterday would yell at me for shaving my head. They were mad because I was different. Then other people started telling me some of the intimate details of their lives. They thought I was handicapped like they were and felt comfortable telling me their problems.

B: So they thought your baldness was due to chemotherapy treatments?

S: Yes. For me, there was the symbolism in shaving your head that you can uncover yourself and be who you are. *GQ* magazine asked me to do an article on the body a few years ago. But they didn't run it because they said it was too serious. I had written it as lightly as I could about why we choose plastic surgery to deny our mortality. Sometimes when hair comes out, and it doesn't matter whether it's related to chemicals or genes, you can uncover your true self or go down the drain. The symbolism of going down the drain is getting a rug. If you want to uncover yourself, you go bald. I'm uncovering who I am.

B: Why the great urge to shave your head? It's not the usual haircut.

S: Of course, to uncover your real self doesn't mean you have to shave your head. I did something symbolically. But I wasn't smart enough to grasp the inner message for a couple of years. I walked around in workshops with a shaved head and then I realized that the message was to uncover feelings on the inside.

B: Why did you wait to shave your head? You had the urge but you didn't act on it for a while.

S: A shaved head isn't very acceptable. My barber wouldn't do it at first. When I said I wanted to do it, people looked at me like I was out of my mind. It wasn't easy to do. It's not like I was some teenager acting crazy during a college football game.

B: So how did you finally do it?

S: I sat and had a regular haircut. As the barber cut it, I said go shorter. I said do more. I kept doing that. And after a while, it was so short, down to about a quarter of an inch, that finally he said, "You might as well shave it all off."

B: And how do you do it now?

S: I shave it with a razor. I'm used to doing this, because as a surgeon, you shave people for surgery.

B: Do you ever cut yourself?

S: I nick it once in a while if I'm in a hurry. It's annoying.

B: So upon acquiring a shaved head, you got a new look.

S: I didn't do it for a look. I did it for an inner need. Once it was done, my wife liked it. It was nice to touch and as warm as a baby's bottom. Our daughter said it was easier to find me in the movies.

B: Some men with shaved heads say that people view them differently, maybe as a little more powerful or sinister.

S: I work with a lot of people who've been ill. They didn't see it as sinister. The so-called normal people did. But the ones with afflictions thought, "This guy's in trouble, too." It worked. There are also people who act like nothing's different. Lots of kids come into my office, too. One kid said, "Look at that guy, he's bald." And the parent said, "Shhhh, don't notice." I'm standing right there and I say, "Your kid is more normal than you are."

B: You have to feel different physically with a shaved head.

S: You notice how cold it is, and that first year, I really had to protect it.

B: How about in the sun?

S: I may put some lotion on it, but I'm outside a lot, running, so it's toughened up. Plus I have good skin.

B: Having such a healthy attitude probably means you've probably never had an urge to get a hairpiece.

S: Never. It would be false and that wouldn't be me. But I once grew a mustache, and it was like there was a stranger in the bathroom. Who's that? I'd ask. Well, it was me.

B: How much hair would you have if you didn't shave?

S: I'd look like most people, with hair on the sides and a bald spot in the middle.

B: With the way you look now, are people more likely to talk to the top of your head than directly into your eyes?

S: No. Now people notice my eyes more. Without hair, your face is colorless. I have blue eyes and people now look so intensely into my eyes that I think they're looking through me. Without hair, there's nothing to distract people. I also look younger without any hair because I don't get gray hair. I look ageless.

B: Did you ever get the sense that your surgical patients might have been more comfortable with a hairy doctor?

S: No. And I point out to students that if you care for people it doesn't matter what you look like. If you care, you're beautiful.

B: Hair matters far too much in our society, doesn't it?

S: It's a cosmetic factor related to aging. Current youth doesn't want to get old so they try to deny their mortality. You spend millions on things. We have four sons. One is concerned about his hair. He can have drugs or surgery. My statement is if you have self-esteem it doesn't matter how many hairs you have on your head.

B: That's beautiful.

Y. A. TITTLE

I'VE LOOKED LIKE I'M SIXTY-THREE SINCE I WAS TWENTY-THREE

Name: Y. A. Tittle
Occupation: Former quarterback, San Francisco 49ers and New York Giants; now an insurance broker
Started Balding: Twenty-one
Minoxidil Opinion: No
Toupee Opinion: It ain't him, babe

BALDMAN: Sports is such a youth-oriented world, where hair equals youth. Was your self-image hurt by being a young bald athlete?

TITTLE: I think so. At a young age, I lost my hair, probably starting in my junior year in college. I'd say it was a source of embarrassment. Everybody else had hair. I was just a junior and everybody had hair. I lost some confidence over it. It was a problem.

B: Was the loss a quick one?

T: It wasn't a drawn-out process. I lost it between the end of one football season and Easter the next year.

B: Boy, that's quick. It went that fast. What was it like before?

T: It was a full head of brownish, reddish hair.

B: What was the family reaction?

T: None. I was off in LSU. But my father was bald and so were my uncles.

B: Did you ever figure, you're a Tittle man, and the hair's gonna leave some day soon?

T: It never entered my mind until it started to fall out. But I sure felt self-conscious once it did.

B: Did anything turn you toward accepting the hair loss?

T: As I got older, got married, had two or three children, it didn't bother me quite as much. I didn't have to worry about

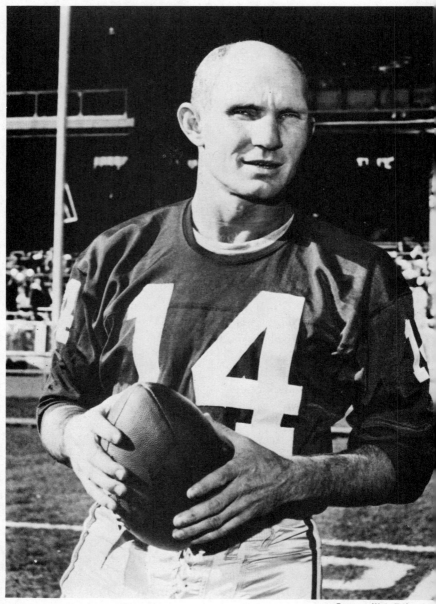

Courtesy of Y. A. Tittle

being in the girl market. I felt less and less self-conscious as I reached thirty. But getting married helped.

B: At what age did you get married?

T: Twenty-one.

B: Your wife must be an incredibly intelligent and fine person not to feel the way men think women will react to a young bald man.

T: Well, I knew her from high school. It never bothered her. Maybe it did, but I didn't know about it.

B: Locker rooms being what they are, your bald head must have been the target for jokes.

T: Nobody in football really gave me a needle. Not my teammates. Opponents? No. You just feel self-conscious. If you're a junior and you're going bald, you're self-conscious.

B: Some would say that being bald young made you more mature.

T: At that time, I always thought of it as a hindrance.

B: What about any ribbing you got in the pros? Did you get any nicknames?

T: Well, the Bald Eagle.

B: You were on the Giants at the same time as kicker Don Chandler. Did you ever hear that he was nicknamed "The Hairless Bunny"?

T: No.

B: Did baldness create problems with your head and your helmet? Did the helmet stick to your head?

T: No, not at all.

B: So your attitude is that you never really enjoyed being bald. Why didn't you ever go for a cover-up?

T: I didn't want to. I'd feel phony. To me, I could not have played football, or any other sports and every afternoon take my hairpiece off in front of my teammates. It would put me in the position of not being the real Y. A. Tittle. If I were away, away from my friends, it might have been different.

B: When minoxidil came out, did people say, "Hey, Y. A., you should try this"?

T: I asked about it. But it's for people who've just started to lose it. I'm not vain enough to use it to regain some hair. That's why I wouldn't wear a hairpiece. But if there were something guaranteed to grow hair, I'd use it. If it were a gradual process, I'd try it.

B: Can you think of any advantage to being bald?

T: I've looked the same every day since I was twenty-one. Everybody's hobbling around and me, I'm going into my prime. I tell everybody I've looked sixty-three since I was twenty-three. What do some of the other people you've talked to think about being bald?

B: Well, people like Joe Garagiola revel in it and make jokes about it.

T: I guess if you have a good, outgoing personality, it helps. I always felt badly about making first impressions. I wanted to wear a cap when I was introduced to someone for the first time. But I was never the type of person who wanted to stand out. And being bald makes you stand out. People know who the bald guy is.

B: Does being bald help you in the insurance business?

T: I'd say the appearance of age gives an experienced feeling to people. I'm not saying baldness does. But baldness does make you look a little older and more mature, and in the insurance business, you need age and experience, and maybe a bald head gives you that. It doesn't hurt you.

B: And finally, how long does it take you to get a haircut?

T: Oh, they just fiddle around my hair the way they always have. They just spend their time asking football questions.

KEN HOWARD

WHY CAN'T I JUST BE MYSELF?

Name: Ken Howard
Occupation: Actor
Started Balding: Early thirties
Minoxidil Opinion: Wouldn't try it
Toupee Opinion: Only wears it professionally and reluctantly

Note: Ken Howard was granted special dispensation to be anointed a Patron Saint because of the achievement attained by appearing in a major television role on Murder, She Wrote, *without the hairpiece he'd worn on other series like* Dynasty *and* The White Shadow. *He admits that Hollywood imposes the hairpiece on him. In real life, he never puts one on. Praise Yul.*

BALDMAN: Congratulations on being Patron Saint and doffing your hairpiece recently in *Murder, She Wrote*.

HOWARD: I never wear a hairpiece in real life. When I created *The White Shadow*, my hair was thinning. The character was a former pro basketball player in his thirties, and I didn't look like a former pro being bald. So I started with the hairpiece then. Whenever I'd show up for lunch or a meeting with a director, my agent would say "Have the hair because this is a romantic leading man." "Yeah, sure, whatever you want." I was always relieved when someone said we like you the way you are.

After a while, it became a symbol of what people actually wanted from me. If the baldness didn't matter, I knew they wanted an interesting person. If they did, they wanted me as some version of a glamourpuss.

I actually started out with a full head of hair but I wore a wig when I played Thomas Jefferson in *1776* on Broadway and then in the film. So I had this auburn thing on my head.

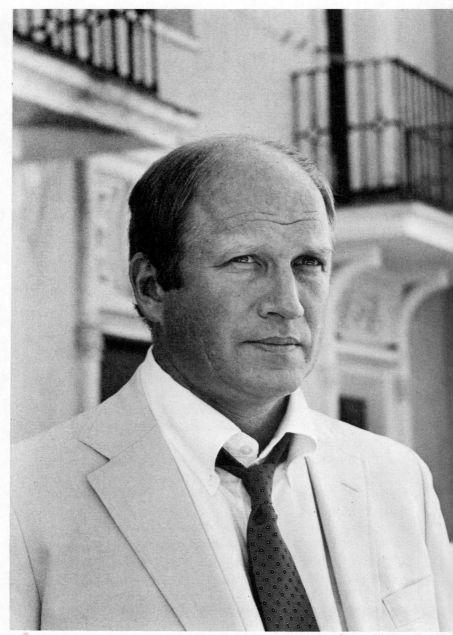

I always found it an irony that this role gave me my first shot and I had hair but didn't get to use it. That was in 1969.

B: When did you start losing it?

H: Because of my father being bald, I figured it was in the cards. I guess I was always aware of it. I had a pretty full head of hair until I was thirty. But I remember the makeup guy started darkening it, so I knew it was starting to go. Then I started doing *The White Shadow*, and wearing a hairpiece sort of made sense. If it were one of those shows that went on forever, I'd be playing it this way, bald.

B: You have the perfect attitude of bald acceptance, which makes me wonder if you feel ridiculous wearing a hairpiece.

H: No, because it's acting. I've put on funny noses. It's fine. As long as it wasn't in real life. There were times when someone would ask me to go attend this particular thing with hair. And I'd go through the real world wearing it and feel like a jerk.

I play golf all the time. Out at Riviera I met a guy who had a very good hairpiece. Guys like us, we can spot 'em. This was a good one. Salt and pepper. So we're out playing. Usually, when I'm out there, I wear a cap and then take it off to get a little sun on my pate. Then he said to me, "Weren't you the guy on this show?" I said yes. Then a couple of weeks later, I see this guy and he's bald as an eagle. One of his buddies told me, "You know, you changed his life. He said that this guy's an actor and he's not wearing his hair on the golf course, so why the hell am I wearing it?"

I feel funny with it in life. In fact, there were a few times where I had to go someplace, and when I appeared, it was best to wear it. So I'd have it in my pocket. I'd walk in like me, go into makeup, and put on this little sheitle and I'd go. As soon as it was over, I'd put it back in my pocket.

B: Because of your blond coloring, losing your hair doesn't seem a big contrast. You don't look any older without your hairpiece.

H: That's part of it. The funny thing is, I've always thought of bald guys as tougher. Where that comes from I don't know.

I remember Otto Preminger, my first director, would shave his head while he was talking to you. With an electric razor. He'd run his hand over his head to see if there were any stubble.

B: You've worked with Charlton Heston. Ever see him without his hairpiece?

H: Nobody in the world has. I don't know if his wife has.

B: Your mother-in-law is Ann Landers. Have you had any problems dealing with being bald that you sought counsel from her?

H: No, not really. Honestly, a lot had to do with my father. He was a big guy who had a hundred funny lines about it. He was a distinguished fellow, a Wall Street guy. It was what he was. I always thought that's who I was going to be. If I had a family of brothers and a father with big shocks of hair, I'd say, "What happened to me?"

B: So you've never had a problem in being bald personally?

H: Absolutely. When I did *Dynasty* and *The Colbys*, if I was going to go to a restaurant at lunch, I'd take off this little doily on my head, put it in my pocket, wipe the makeup off my face and go. Then I'd come back up. That's the way it was. It was always makeup to me.

B: Do they make hairpieces for you on the sets?

H: There's a guy named Ziggy. He's great. He can make one that's not real hair, that you can wash in cold water and Woolite, believe it or not, then you can shake it out and stick it on. I always find a way to make sure somebody pays for it. It's a point of pride. If you don't pay for it, I don't have to wear it.

B: How many hairpieces do you have now?

H: I don't have any right now, because now I have this part in *Murder, She Wrote.* I don't need anything now. When I get called upon to do something, I just come in au naturel. I haven't done that much where it was all that way. But I may have one piece stuck away somewhere.

B: Is there something wrong in our society that hair is such an obsessive focus?

H: I'll tell you my pet theory. The one thing that separates the human race from the rest of the animal kingdom is we know we're going to die. Never have people been so scared of it as in this day and age as it is now and in America. Everything's about death. Liposuction, tummy tucks, hairpieces. I want to take care of myself and be healthy, but I've gone the other way. I'd like to live to a ripe old age and have a good time. So I'm getting older and this is another example of it. I'm all for it.

B: I feel like applauding but both my hands are busy.

H: You are going to die. Accept it.

B: Yes. Yes. I must applaud. Say, who wears rotten toupees in Hollywood?

H: As you know, there are some gorgeous, sexy women walking around that guys are crazy about who have very petite busts. They have long legs and tight asses. They know they're ideal women for a lot of men. Then with some women, it's a big issue. "Oh, my god? how can I go through life without big breasts?" and they go to a doctor. For some guys, whatever hair they have works out fine. For others, it's symbolic of everything.

B: About those bad toupees.

H: Well, you know, what's worse than a bad toupee are the guys who comb it over from their left ears. They're hysterical. What I really loved was Zero Mostel. He'd lick three hairs and comb it from the back. It was part of his nutty image.

B: When you saw the news about minoxidil, did others suggest you try it?

H: All the time. But I have every intention of going to my grave the way I came in, with whatever scars, warts and bags I have.

B: In *Dynasty*, did the producers think the Diahann Carroll character wouldn't have slept with a bald guy?

H: It wasn't even discussed. But I'm not an idiot. When a guy named Garrett Boydston is your part, there you go. You wear it. It's not like someone twisted my arm. If he'd been written a different way, with something else to the character, I'd go for it. Diahann would have been the first to say, "Go for it."

B: Any other bald stories?

H: When I did *Seesaw* on Broadway in the spring of 1973, I was referred to as Mayor Lindsay's lookalike. I was tall and in a suit. Then I left to do *Adam's Rib*. My hair was thinning, but not so you'd know it on stage. The fellow who replaced me on *Seesaw* was John Gavin, and we went out to lunch and Gavin said, "I can see your hair is thinning on top. Like mine. I have this little piece I'm going to wear onstage. The guy who made it is Ziggy. He's the best. You clip it on and it's no big deal. When you're a little older, it's something you can use when you're a leading man." Years later, when he became ambassador to Mexico, he made a point of saying, "I'm not acting now, so never mind with the hairpiece."

B: Do most people on a set or in a show know you're wearing a piece?

H: Sure, I unclip it and put it in my pocket.

B: Did the boys on *White Shadow* kid you about it and play with it?

H: Yeah, sure, some, but I was in on the joke. That's one of the things. People can kid you about it if they know you truly don't give a damn.

B: Have you been insulted because you're bald?

H: I remember one time. I was sitting in a bar in New York after doing a show. A pretty quiet bar. A very elegant bar. I sat there just to have a cold beer. I have my doily in my pocket, which I was wearing in the show I was doing. A Neil Simon show. This dame, who's probably my age, was three sheets to the wind, a little blowsy. Maybe she realized the guy she was with wouldn't take her home for the night. She started with me. She said, "Hello, big guy," like, "Hello, sailor." She was real friendly. Then she put her hand on my arm. I just said, "I'm here having a beer on my way home." I tried to get rid of her. Then it got to the point where I tried to excuse myself, and then I said to the bartender, "I don't want to be rude, but could you help me out here, I just want to get out." So at that point, she turns around and says, "Excuse me," and something like "you're a jerk—and you're bald." Then she walked away. I felt like saying, "I may be bald, but I bet I'm going to get laid tonight and you're not."

I told that to my lovely wife, and she patted me on the head and said, "Good for you, honey."

B: Your lovely wife has never minded your being bald?

H: Obviously not. As a matter of fact, if I had any self-consciousness about it, it was the other way, like, "Why can't I just be myself?"

B: It's a pity that when they look for a distinguished senatorial type, they don't think of a bald guy.

H: Well, it depends how old. If it's an older age group, it's okay. But it depends on how you're perceived. It's also the tone of the piece. If it's *Rage of Angels*, and it's glitzy and opposite Jaclyn Smith, there isn't that much texture. You wear it.

B: But my point is it's people's perception that Jaclyn Smith wouldn't be caught dead having a bald leading man.

H: Right. That's true.

B: Do you think we're viewed as second-class citizens?

H: Only in the silly part of the world. When I was lecturing at Harvard, I didn't think I needed the hairpiece. If you run a company, you don't need it. Or to be a military officer or coach a team. But to be an actor, you're already suspect. So you have to go along with it.

B: Do your students who thought of you as a haired person express surprise when seeing you're bald?

H: There was some humor here and there. But it's part of who I am.

B: (Applause.) Ken Howard, you are a great bald man.

H: One of the running jokes people hit me with is this. When people see me, they don't realize how big I am. The notion, and this comes from other bald guys, they say, "You've got it easy because nobody can see the top of your head."

B: Yeah. Sure.

H: There's some truth to that in the regular world. People would say, "You're not so bald." "Oh, yes, I am," I say, "wait until I sit down." One thing that irritates me is when a guy who's fifty starts talking about how he's really concerned about his little bald spot. Oh come on, give me a break. You've gotten this far, you should only know. I respond to any jokes about hair.

B: I hope you'll join me in the Baldness Anti-Defamation League.

H: Well, I'm pleased and honored to be in your opus.

B: You are a beautiful Patron Saint.

H: You know, this part I have with *Murder, She Wrote* might be a series, so I can be an ongoing Patron Saint.

B: Will you walk around during the series with the hairpiece in your pocket?

H: If this series is a hit, I'll never need it again. Say, who's your number-one Patron Saint?

B: Yul Brynner.

H: Ah, yes, but to me the number one is Sean Connery. After James Bond, he said he'd never wear the bloody thing again.

He used to have it in his pocket. He never wore it on the golf course. He was happy to get away from it and I always had that in the back of my mind.

B: God bless him.

WILLARD SCOTT

BALDNESS IS LIKE A BROTHERHOOD, LIKE TWO GUYS PASSING EACH OTHER ON HARLEYS

Name: Willard Scott
Occupation: Weatherman, the *Today Show*
Started Balding: Twenty
Toupee Opinion: Only for fun or if advertisers demand it
Time for Haircut: Twelve minutes

BALDMAN: Is God bald?

SCOTT: (Laughs.) Well, being a Christian, I look at the Trinity. Jesus has an awful lot of hair and a beard. But he was thirty-three years old. If we had a later picture of him . . .

B: He might be receding?

S: Yeah. But I'd also think God would have something on his head to denote that he's God, like a crown or some magnificent cape, so we might not know if he's bald.

B: When did you come to the *Today Show*?

S: Ten years ago in March.

B: So that was a few years after Joe Garagiola left. Do you think that in those fallow years between bald stars of the show, the program went downhill?

S: Well, Bill Monroe was there [delivering the news from Washington]. But I just think if you hire a bald man, he brings you luck.

B: When did you start losing your hair?

S: About twenty. That's typical of people who lose their hair because of heredity. It came from my mother's side.

B: Grandfather and uncles bald?

S: Yeah, almost to a person. In college, I started going very thin. By the time I was twenty-one, I had a bald spot. Now, when I get a hairpiece, I have to get a complete piece because I don't have enough hair to tuck it into.

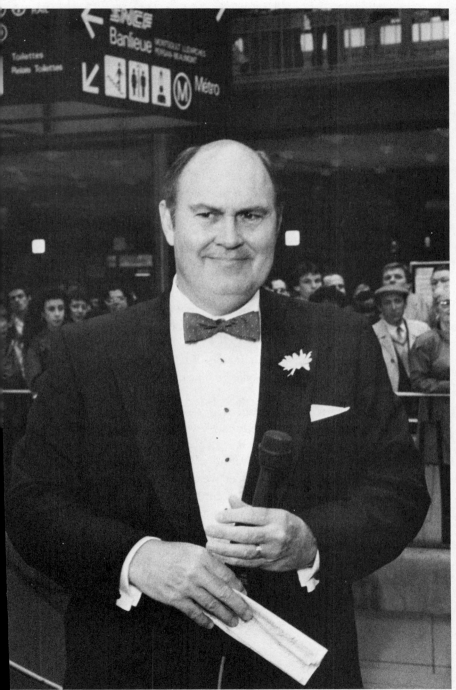

B: Was that a new one I saw you wearing the other day?

S: A brand-new one. It's a full piece. You can't tell it's fake. I'd even wear that one to church. No one would know.

B: It does look more natural.

S: I think it does. With the old one, you could really see it was fake. But you can't see it with this one. He gave me more hair with this one. From the back, the old one looked like some big plop sitting there.

B: You've said frequently that you wear it for fun. But isn't it also a little poking of fun at the people who say you have to cover up?

S: No, it's purely for fun. There's never been any pressure to wear it. The reason I started wearing it is that I was doing a commercial for a guy who didn't like baldheaded people. Ever since, I've worn it like an option. There's an agency guy who calls and says he has some clients who want hair, some others who don't. The cranberry people don't want hair.

B: So generally, you wear it inside, but go natural outside.

S: It never leaves New York. It's just a fun piece. It's really nothing.

B: Well, if it's really nothing, why wear it?

S: For the agencies and advertisers who want me to wear it— and the fact that I can take it off. It's a conversation piece. It's a hype. That's why. Otherwise, there's nothing to it. I never take it home. I never wear it anywhere else. It stays up in New York on a form. I get ten or twenty calls per week from people who ask me about wearing hairpieces. That's because I'm so easy and free about wearing it or not. I never make fun of it or anybody who wears one.

B: But you have to admit that some people wear really bad ones.

S: Oh, some are atrocious. I wore some for the fifteen or twenty-five years that I've worn hair. You have to find someone who cares about you and will take time to work with you. In the beginning, I got a hairpiece that the guy wouldn't even cut for me. He said go to your barber and have him cut it for you. It was really a cop-out. He really didn't like the end result and didn't want to be responsible. Once you cut it, you can't put it back.

B: How do you feel you look, bald versus haired?

S: No difference. People recognize me with it or without it.

B: Do bald guys come up to you for advice?

S: All the time. It's almost like a brotherhood, like people who pass each other on Harleys. It's simpatico. You're just one of the group. I was down in Florida in a parking lot and a guy sticks his head out of his car and pats his head and points to me. Bald people know each other that way.

B: Do you hear much about antibaldness prejudice?

S: I never hear any of it. I've never felt it. I feel being bald has been an advantage. Most bald people I know are aggressive, very dynamic people. There's the old gag about not wasting your hormones on your head. I think there's something to it. I can't think of a bald guy who isn't an extrovert. Look at Danny DeVito.

B: But there is the Silent Baldority out there who wonder, "Why me?"

S: I've never run into that. I might annoy them a little by what I do with mine. But I feel just the opposite. I think it's great. I have fun with being bald. Some people think it's a real macho thing not to have hair.

B: What would be your advice to bald men on how to fully accept their pate's fate?

S: That's a difficult question because I don't have any problem with it at all. I've never met a bald man who didn't accept it. If a man feels because he doesn't have hair that it cuts back on his virility or his ability to forge ahead, that's sad.

B: Were you married young?

S: Yeah, but I'd lost most of my hair by then.

B: So your wife didn't mind?

S: Oh, I think women find baldness very attractive. I've never known it to be a detriment. Just the opposite. Most bald-headed people have incredible personalities. Look at it from this angle: if you're so hung up on appearances, you may lack substance. But the bald person depends a lot more on personality than looks.

B: You depend heavily on your personality.

S: Yeah, for 90 percent. I have no illusions of grandeur. I'm fifty-five and overweight. But I'm telling you, women love bald heads.

B: They come up and want to touch yours?

S: They come right over.

B: Philosophically, do you think men who shave all their hair off should be considered bald? Telly Savalas says he doesn't consider himself bald.

S: That's surprising. I think he just didn't want to fool with the look. I've gotta believe he's proud of it or he wouldn't have done it. It made him a character. I don't think it's a negative. It's a positive and Telly's the classic example.

B: One last thing. How long does it take you to get a haircut?

S: About twelve minutes.

B: That much time?

S: Well, we talk a lot.

LOUIS GOSSETT, JR.

THE SHAVED HEAD IS SOME KIND OF SEXUAL STIMULANT

Name: Louis Gossett, Jr.
Occupation: Film and television actor, known for his roles in
Roots, *An Officer and a Gentleman* and *Sadat*
Started Balding: Eighteen
Minoxidil Opinion: Never heard of it
Toupee Opinion: Personally, it's a cheat
Time for shave: Six minutes

BALDMAN: You shave your head. When did that start?

GOSSETT: I did it when I was doing the film of *The River Niger*. I was playing the part of James Earl Jones's doctor friend who was supposed to be fifty-five. I wasn't quite that old. This was a really hot summer. It was over 100 degrees every day in L.A. For practical considerations, it just didn't pay to gray my hair and put old-age makeup on my face. It would just sweat off. So I shaved off all my hair, and then grew a little back and made that gray. Then I grew a mustache and beard and let it gray. When I finished the film, I showed up around my agency and all around town, and people thought I looked fantastic. It launched me on a great career. I'm a leading man. But for some TV pilots, they made me put on hair.

B: You're one of the very few bald leading men around.

G: It's true. Originally, for pilots and movies, they had me put on hair—

B: That's terrible.

G: —so that I'd look conventionally handsome.

B: What was the part where the producer finally said, "Okay, we're not going to make him put on hair?"

G: It was probably *The Lazarus Syndrome* [in 1979]. I had a thick mustache and the bald head.

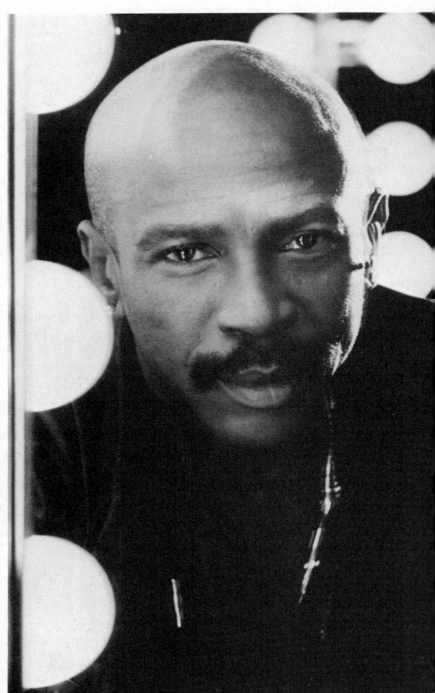

Dick Zimmerman

B: You also wore some hair to play Fiddler in *Roots*.

G: That was a character. The makeup people were happy to start with a bald head and build a character from that. It helped them a lot.

B: When you shaved your hair completely, were you thinking at all of Telly?

G: No, not at all. It would have been a pain in my neck to apply and reapply that makeup in the summer. That's all I was thinking about it. I've worn hair in different things to look different. I had a collection of hairpieces for that purpose. When I shaved it, I had to get full headpieces. I definitely wasn't looking to have hair. My hairline was already receding. But what happened was that shaving it all off expanded my career so I could be more versatile. I can play three, four or five parts in a movie or play.

B: What have we seen recently where you had hair?

G: I let a little hair grow back in a Disney flick called *The Fourth of July*. And I let my natural hair grow back and put hair on top for Sadat because Sadat had a certain look. I would let it grow back for whatever role. I'll let some of it grow back if I get a chance to play Kwame Nkruma.

B: What would you look like if you didn't shave?

G: Like Roscoe Lee Browne. Very thick on the sides. Tufted in the middle with bald spot in the back. It's good. I like it.

B: Which look do you prefer?

G: I like it the way it is. I like shaving. I'm used to it. I call it starting from neutral.

B: What do you shave with?

G: I started using an electric razor, then a razor blade and I cut myself. Then I used a thing called No-Blade, which took too long to do. Now I use a cream depilatory, which comes in a tube, and it takes six minutes. I shave it with a plastic dull-edged razor. It's neat and it's wonderful.

B: The shaved head is often very attractive to women.

G: Well, I was just going to say that. It's very tactile. Women just love it.

B: Any woman do anything particularly odd to your shaved head?

G: I don't know if you want to put it in the book.

B: Sure, why not. If you say it, I'll print it.

G: Use your imagination. It's obviously some kind of sexual stimulant. They want to try all kinds of things.

B: Well, I think I'll go out and get that cream depilatory myself. Do men come up and ask for advice on shaving their heads?

G: Men want to, but they're afraid to do it because they don't know what it would look like. They're afraid that their head won't look good. I got lucky. My head is all right.

B: That's true. You do have a well-shaped head.

G: Just lucky.

B: I've noticed that, unfortunately, your TV series haven't lasted very long. Not one has gone past a season.

G: No, none have.

B: Do you think this is an example of antibaldness bias?

G: No, not at all. Television doesn't want too much quality. Not in this day. There used to be very good television in the Kennedy era.

B: Were you bothered that your bald show was replaced by a show with lots of hair, starring Jaclyn Smith?

G: No, actually, it was replaced by *Kojak*.

B: So it wasn't *Christine Cromwell*?

G: No. When that happened, I sent Telly some flowers, with a note saying, "Well, instead of a negative of the film, it's a positive." He was very touched by that. We have a picture taken when he came to visit me on the set of *The Deep*. It's me, him and a mold of my bald head. Me on one side, head in the middle and Telly on the other side.

B: Telly refused to talk to me because he doesn't think he's bald.

G: Maybe he has some insecurities about it. I call myself a bald man. I am a bald man.

B: And I applaud you for that.

G: I chose to shave it, I got a windfall and I choose to keep it that way.

B: Then you've not felt prejudice in movies and TV against your bald head.

G: There isn't too much of an onus. It's distinctive. Sometimes people mistake me for the guy who plays "Hawk" [Avery Brooks], who has a natural head of hair. I have a feeling I've been copied a lot. I was up for the role in the baseball movie *Major League*, but they couldn't afford me, so they got an actor who shaved his head like me. So I am honored with it. I can play anything.

B: But while you succeed being bald, other bald actors feel the only way they can get ahead is with hairpieces.

G: Well, I'd be lying to the public. It's difficult to wear that hair. I'd have to wear it all the time. It's uncomfortable. It's uncomfortable to kiss a woman and when she runs her hand through your hair, it winds up in her hand. It's a terrible shock.

B: Is that the worst thing that happened to you when you wore a piece?

G: Yeah. Hugging a woman and seeing how shocked she was to find it wasn't my real hair.

B: Oooh, that's awful. You must have been young then.

G: Yes.

B: Women—the women who matter—seem to care a lot less about men balding than men do.

G: It's a male vanity thing. I haven't lost any dates or girlfriends or wives because I have no hair. In fact, some women think it's a sign of virility.

B: If you had to give advice to bald men who are unhappy being bald, what would you say?

G: Well, there's the standard thing that hair doesn't grow on a busy street. But it's beyond baldness. It's the soul inside. It's the spirit. You develop who you are to the best of your abilities.

B: When you lost your hair naturally, did you want to cover up in any way?

G: Sure. I wore hairpieces. But they didn't feel like me. I was a little bitter because it fell out so early, when I was eighteen or nineteen.

B: How old were you when you accepted it?

G: About twenty-five.

B: Did your family give you support?

G: I got a lot of support from my friends. They were actors and they said, "You're still a fine actor."

B: Do you care about things like minoxidil?

G: What's that?

B: The drug that purports to grow hair.

G: I don't pay attention to any of that.

B: That's wonderful. Hey, you've got a perfect attitude.

G: I know medically that there's no real thing to grow hair the way you want it. I don't mind shaving the two or three times a week I need to. Men have to shave their face every day.

B: So you're happy with the way you are and that way is bald.

G: I am.

B: Well, clearly, you are a Patron Saint of Baldness.

G: (Laughs.) Thanks.

NEWS FLASH! TELLY SAVALAS DOESN'T THINK HE'S
BALD ... THAT'S WHY THIS GREAT PATRON SAINT OF
BALDNESS WON'T TALK TO ME

Amazing but true, isn't it? The baldo di tutti baldi won't talk to
me. Incomprehensible!

Not since the advent of Yul Brynner in the 1940s has a fully
bald man captured the imagination of the world as Telly Savalas
has. When his hair-breaking series, *Kojak*, made its debut on
October 24, 1973, the world changed a little. The image of the
strong, macho detective, heretofore aggressively haired, had been
altered to accommodate Telly Savalas, a fully shaved, lollypop-
sucking New York City detective who went around saying, "Who
loves ya, baby?" He made women purr and men cower. He
intimidated, charmed and overwhelmed. Men who imitated Telly
were automatically nicknamed "Kojak."

Even though he seemed to run roughshod over his colleagues—
particularly the overhaired Detective Stavros, played by Telly's
brother, George—they respected him. They never forgot that
Kojak was a damned good detective and a fair boss. (Keen dome
observers will remember the balding Kevin Dobson as another
detective—"Crocker!" Kojak would roar—in his prehairpiece,
pre–*Knots Landing* period.)

Kojak lasted five seasons on CBS and returned in 1989 on
ABC. In the interim, no bald star completely filled the unhaired
vacuum. No one seemed to be able to parlay his bare scalp into
full-blown, prime-time stardom. There were some pretenders,
like Gerald McRaney (of *Simon and Simon* and *Major Dad*), Bob
Newhart, William Conrad (of *Cannon*) and Michael Conrad (of
Hill Street Blues). But nobody, absolutely nobody, did it better
than the terrific Telly.

Telly wasn't always perfectly bald. In the 1950s, he was a
hairy State Department official and ABC News executive. Then
the acting bug hit him. He started his new career with abundant

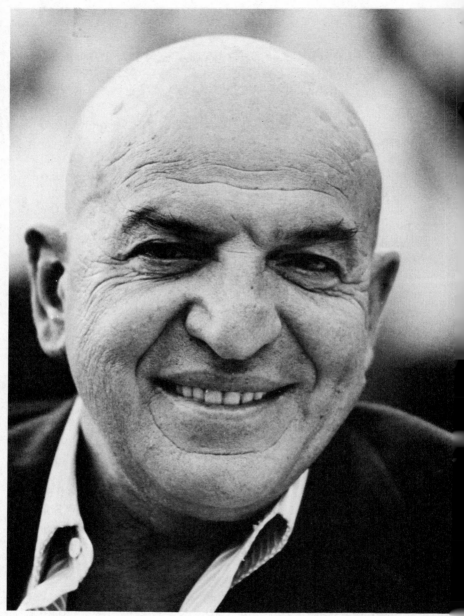

hair, and you can see him that way in *The Birdman of Alcatraz* and *Cape Fear*.

Then, to appear as Pontius Pilate, the cruel Roman governor who refused to save Jesus from the crucifix in the George Stevens epic, *The Greatest Story Ever Told*, Telly shaved his head for good. And he has shaved it every day since, lest it return as bushels of lush Greek curls.

For twenty-five years now, Telly has been the bald man's bald man. Yet he insists that he's not truly bald and won't talk about being bald. He won't talk about being the shining example of bald saintliness, a beacon for any of us who doubt the manly value of our bare pates.

No, Telly really won't come forth to tell us how being bald changed his life.

I came across this bizarre twist in my odyssey through the bald world through correspondence with Telly's publicist, Mike Mamakos. I wrote two letters to Telly and then Mike and I twice discussed why Telly wouldn't talk. Here's how it went. To begin, excerpts from my first letter.

Dear Mr. Savalas,

I want to take this brief moment of your time to persuade you to talk to me for *Bald Like Me*, the book on baldness I am currently writing. I know you've told Mr. Mamakos that you didn't want to do it. But please, hear me out, because having you in the book would mean so much.

Mr. Mamakos told me that because you shave your head every day you do not consider yourself truly bald. I understand that. But I'm sure you realize that people consider you the most evolved form of male baldness. You are a Patron Saint of Baldness, not only because you look so good bald, but because you had the good taste to purposely shave your head, while the rest of us have to wait for nature to take its damned time.

Bald Like Me is a celebration of baldness. Sure, it has a point of view—against the merchants of fakery, who would put false hair on top of our scalps—because, Mr. Savalas, most of us ordinary bald folk are treated as second-class citizens. We're told we're less sexy, less virile, less youthful and less acceptable in our society because we are less of hair. We need a manifesto of bald rights!

In TV, for instance, there are very few positive images of bald men. Besides yourself, Carl Reiner, Charles Kuralt, Lou Gossett, Jr., and a handful of others, bald men are portrayed as evil (Danny DeVito in *Taxi*), near-sighted and out of control ("Mr. Magoo"), fat and sloppy (William Conrad in anything), offensive (Don Rickles), sexually neuter (Bob Newhart in both his sitcoms), a backwoods boob (Sorrell Booke as Boss Hogg in *The Dukes of Hazzard*), bizarre (Jackie Coogan as Uncle Fester in *The Addams Family*) and bestial-but-kindly (Bull in *Night Court*, played by Richard Moll, who also shaves his head).

As for my need for you, Mr. Savalas, I can only say that you are the greatest positive image of baldness in our country today.

For you, a bare head enhances your looks, or I assume that you wouldn't have decided to shave your hair off. Women often remark on your sexiness, and I'm sure your "look" has helped you in your life. I think your views on hairlessness, why you decided to embrace baldness, and what life was like for you with hair, would be of interest to people naturally losing their hair— or those who would like to shave it all off.

I'd really like you to think about this. You certainly have no reason to want to do any favor for me. After all, you don't know me. But think of the millions of men who find the inexorable recession of their hair psychologically unbearable. They need some inspiration and some humor. They need to be told they're just as good as a fully haired man. You, among others, would greatly help that healing process.

Now that was a friendly letter, wasn't it? I guarantee that Telly had never met anyone who was going to ask the questions

I was going to ask. ("Have you ever been denied housing because you were bald, Mr. Savalas?") But Mr. Mamakos, a very good protector of his client, demurred. Here is a reconstruction of that conversation:

> *Mike:* I'm sorry. Telly's gonna pass.
>
> *Me:* Why?
>
> *Mike:* He's quite vehement on the subject. He doesn't think of himself as bald. He's not congenitally bald. Every morning he shaves his head. So he's not naturally bald.
>
> *Me:* But if he shaves his head every day, then, naturally, he's bald.
>
> *Mike:* If he didn't shave it every day, he'd have a full head of hair.
>
> *Me:* Yeah, and if my mother had wheels, she'd be a trolley car. She doesn't, so she's not. Telly's image is that he has no hair, thus he's bald, by hereditary means or not. Listen, Mike, the fact remains that Telly is the best-known bald guy in America if not the world.
>
> *Mike:* I know, I know. But Telly feels he just wouldn't be honest with himself if he talked about being bald. Because he really isn't. It's got something to do with his Greek conscience.
>
> *Me:* C'mon Mike. You and I both know he's bald. It helped his career and perpetuated his image.
>
> *Mike:* I know that and you know that. But Telly doesn't want to talk about it.
>
> *Me:* Okay, what can I do?
>
> *Mike:* Give up.
>
> *Me:* No. What if I send some more pieces of the book? Maybe that will work.
>
> *Mike:* You can try. But he was pretty vehement.

Pretty bizarre, huh? My point here is that it doesn't matter that Telly isn't bald in the hereditary sense. Who cares? To me, it's even better, even more beautiful, that Telly so wanted to be

fully bald, rather than fully haired, that he shaved it all off
and continues to shave it off, so he can be a fully evolved
bald man.

Telly is a Bald Wanna Be! I can hear him saying when the
chance to play Pontius came to him: "I wanna be bald."

And he was!

While I partly respected Telly's statement that he didn't want
to talk, I didn't fully understand why. So I wrote another letter,
with a more pleading tone. I had hoped to prove to Telly that
I was persistent, funny and cognizant of his feelings.

Dear Mr. Savalas,

What can I say? Mike told me that you wanted to pass on
talking to me about baldness. Really, I do respect that decision.
I'm just going to try again to convince you otherwise.

From what Mike said, you seem most sensitive about
discussing baldness when you are not naturally bald. Rest assured
that whatever I write about you, it would note that you would
have a full head of hair if you didn't shave it off every day (and
incidentally, I would love to watch your daily shaving routine,
just for the sport of it).

But I must repeat my previous assertion that by participating
in my book, *Bald Like Me*, you would help some other sensitive
bald men accept their state. Because you are a bald demigod
(even if you attained that status with shaving cream and razor),
and have succeeded in great part because of your very
hairlessness, I believe that you are a true inspiration. This isn't
fawning here, Mr. Savalas. This is truth. If you ask anyone for a
list of three leading bald men, you're on it. And you are lauded,
not criticized for it. Few men get kudos for not having hair. You
do. Your baldness is as important to you as a mustache was to
Clark Gable or a cigar to George Burns. It is part of your image,
no doubt about it. You are living proof that people don't need
to seek solace in toupees, weaves, transplants or minoxidil to
feel better about their hair loss. They can feel as good about

themselves as you obviously do, even if you are bald by choice. And in fact, a prochoice baldie is so important to me. You're one of those rare guys who *wanted* to be bald, and you prove this each and every day of your life. All hail Telly's razor!!!

Because of your special prochoice baldie status, I'd naturally ask different questions of you than someone who lost their hair naturally. I'd concentrate on the positive effect it has had on your personal life and career, not on the angst it might have caused you, an area of examination I explore with so-called natural baldies.

I know you may think I am maddeningly persistent. And I guess I am. I'm a reporter by nature. But I'm a man on a mission. You don't have to feel that mission in order to agree to a short interview with me. I hope you agree. As an extra added bonus to another amusing letter, I've attached my ever-growing list of baldness quotations. I hope you enjoy it.

Given what Mike said was your vehemence about not participating in my project, I'm not sure any of this will change your mind. I honestly hope it does, but I doubt it. Whatever your decision, I would greatly appreciate it if you would call me to talk about it. Maybe my voice and personal persuasion might help me.

Anyway, whatever you decide, I appreciate your time and consideration.

Do you think I sucked up enough? I do. It still didn't get me anywhere and I thought the second letter was pretty damn good. I would have taken the interview gladly even if he wouldn't let me see him shave. I would have taken submitting written questions for his written answers. But no. Telly stood firm. Again, a talk with Mike Mamakos:

Mike: Telly's gonna pass again. But he told me to tell you that he thinks you're very funny and wishes you all the luck in the world with the project.

Me: You know, Mike, I think Telly's making a big stink about a small subject.

Mike: Well, that's just the way he is. But he wishes you his best.

Me: That doesn't do me much good, Mike. Doesn't he realize the station he occupies in the bald world?

Mike: He doesn't think in those terms.

Me: I'm not going to give up. I know he'll be in New York filming new episodes of *Kojak.* I'll find him.

Mike: That's up to you.

I let my pursuit rest for a few months. Then I reached the New York production offices of *Kojak,* and they told me where Telly would be shooting an episode. That Friday, he would be at Hudson Street in Lower Manhattan at 9:00 A.M., supposedly filming at a chemical company building.

Every bald guy I saw quickened my pulse. I thought every large truck that stopped would unload cameras and crewmen. I stood there for three hours. But I never saw Telly and I never saw a *Kojak* crew.

Maybe it was a conspiracy. Maybe they canceled or moved the day's shoot. Maybe bad information.

All I know is the greatest living Bald Patron Saint won't talk to me. Am I mad? Sure. But, Telly, listen up. Who loves your bald head, baby?

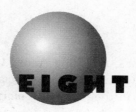

THE BALDIE AWARDS

○

FILM DIVISION

Best Film
Gandhi

**Best Film Unnecessarily Starring a Haired Man
Playing a Real-Life Bald Man**
All That Jazz, starring Roy Scheider as Bob Fosse
(directed by Fosse)

Best Actor
Yul Brynner, *The King and I*

Best Actor Sitting Around without His Hairpiece On
George Burns, *The Sunshine Boys*

**Best Actor Who Proved He Doesn't Have to Wear a
Hairpiece Ever Again if He Doesn't Want to**
Sean Connery, *The Untouchables*

Best Supporting Actor, Comedy
Peter Boyle as the monster (especially when he sang
"Puttin' on the Ritz") in *Young Frankenstein*

Best Supporting Actor, Drama (tie)
Lionel Barrymore, as evil Mr. Potter in *It's a
Wonderful Life,* and
Telly Savalas as Pontius Pilate in *The Greatest Story
Ever Told*

Best Supporting Actor, Shaved Head
Louis Gossett, Jr., *An Officer and a Gentleman*

Best Supporting Actor with Camera Trained Entirely on Shaved Head
Marlon Brando, *Apocalypse Now*

Best Actress
(vacant)

Best Supporting Actress
Persis Khambatta, *Star Trek*

Best Director
Billy Wilder, *Sunset Boulevard*

Best Make-Up for a Legion of Extraterrestrial Baldies
Alien Nation

TELEVISION DIVISION

Best Dramatic Series
Kojak

Best Comedy Series (tie)
The Famous Adventures of Mister Magoo, and
The Phil Silvers Show

Best Actor (Drama)
Edward Asner, *Lou Grant*

Best Actor (Comedy)
Danny DeVito, *Taxi*

Best Actor Who Wished He Didn't Have to Wear a Hairpiece (Drama)
Ken Howard, *The White Shadow*

Best Actor Who Kept Failing at Series after Series
Tim Conway, star of *The Tim Conway Show, The Tim Conway Show, The Tim Conway Comedy Hour* and *Rango*

Best Actor Who Can Walk on Water
Gavin MacLeod, *The Love Boat*

Best Actress
(vacant)

Best Supporting Actor (tie)
William Frawley, *I Love Lucy,* and
Werner Klemperer, *Hogan's Heroes*

Best Supporting Actor Taking Abuse from Another Bald Actor (Comedy)
Richard Deacon as Mel Cooley in *The Dick Van Dyke Show,* who withstood a withering barrage of invective from Carl Reiner, playing Alan Brady

Best Supporting Actor Who Suffered No Lasting Ill Effects from the Embarrassment of Wearing a Hairpiece in a Single Episode
Alan Rachins, *L.A. Law*

Best Supporting Actor, Shaved Head
Richard Moll, *Night Court*

Best Supporting Actor, Perfectly Round Head
Jackie Coogan, *The Addams Family*

Best Supporting Actor Losing the Most Hair during the Course of a Series
Rob Reiner, *All in the Family*

Best Bald Supporting Actor Replacing Another Bald Actor (Comedy)
Richard Deacon replacing Roger C. Carmel in *The Mothers-in-Law*

Best Children's Show Producer-Director
Yul Brynner, *Life with Snarky Parker*

Best Writer
Carl Reiner, *The Dick Van Dyke Show* and *Your Show of Shows*

SPECIAL BALDIE BROTHERHOOD AWARDS

Comedy Series Friendliest to the Bald
All in the Family, featuring Rob Reiner, Sherman Hemsley, Mel Stewart, Bill Quinn, Burt Mustin

Dramatic Series Friendliest to the Bald
Hill Street Blues, featuring
Michael Conrad, Rene Enriquez, Bob Prosky, Jeffrey
Tambor and George Wyner

Mini-Series Friendliest to the Bald
Roots, featuring
John Amos, Louis Gossett, Jr., Moses Gunn, Edward
Asner and Scatman Crothers

Producer Friendliest to the Bald
Norman Lear, the aggressively bald creator of
*All in the Family, Maude, The Jeffersons, Diff'rent
Strokes, One Day at a Time* and *Mary Hartman, Mary
Hartman,*
which, in total, featured sixteen bald actors at one
time or another

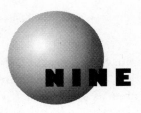

NINE

UPJOHN: THE EVIL EMPIRE
OF MINOXIDIL

○

My boyfriend has spent six months putting minoxidil on his
head. He's got tits, but I don't see any hair yet.
—COMEDIAN ELAYNE BOOSLER

ON THE DAY I left to face the Darth Vaders of Baldness at
Upjohn and the hairy elves who churn out minoxidil, a man's
blond toupee flew off right before my eyes. It was a windy day
in Manhattan, and as the youngish man walked toward me, I
saw it come off its moorings. First it flut-flut-fluttered, then it
whipped backward off his head, blowing end-over-end down the
Avenue of the Americas. I last saw it going south, with him
running madly in pursuit.

Then there was this headline and story from the *New York*
Post: "COPS: BALDIE FLIPS WIG, TRIES TO KILL HAIR-
CLINIC BOSS." A Bronx man, obsessed with going bald and
receiving minoxidil treatments at a Long Island clinic, became
convinced that the drug had created a heart condition. Not only
that, it hadn't grown any hair. It was hard to know which tragedy
sent him over the line. But he wanted revenge. So he barged
into the clinic, wielding a handgun and a knife. He tried to
shoot two men, including one clinic worker, and then tried to
slash them. The man was subdued, and in the hoop-de-do, his
toupee came off. A detective concluded, "The rug was on the
rug."

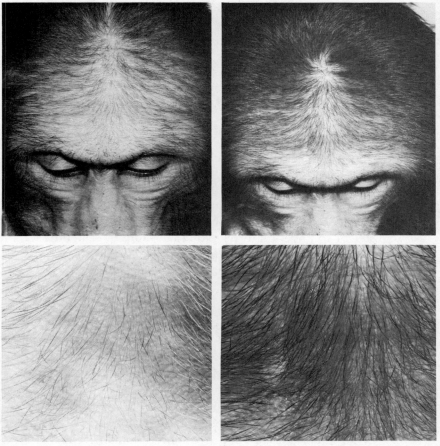

This is a minoxidil monkey, a stump-tailed macaque, forced against his will to have Upjohn's drug swabbed on his balding forehead. First he was balding (top left), then he had minoxidil treatments (top right), then the treatments stopped and the new hair fell out (bottom left), and finally the treatments resumed (bottom right). If he wants a full head of hair, he must use minoxidil for the rest of his life. Will it make a difference in his social life? Will he get a better job? What is a monkey to do?   *Courtesy of Dr. Hideo Uno*

I believe that Bronx Baldie's aim—in gaining a measure of revenge on a medication that is not very effective—was true. Unfortunately, his execution was off the mark. We can't, tempting as it may be, arm a vigilante militia to take up arms against the hairmeisters. We can only raise our domes with pride and hope somebody notices.

These pretrip tales told me that the pates of the Bald Gods were shining upon me, blessing my trip to Kalamazoo in the name of the Silent Baldority. This was not going to be an ordinary trip. I needed to know more about the people behind the demonic minoxidil. Like Marlow in Joseph Conrad's *Heart of Darkness*, who sought to understand the evil around him by searching for Kurtz, the mysterious and reclusive Congo trader, I embarked on a quest to understand the haired evil surrounding me.

Kalamazoo, Michigan, is a city of eighty thousand known for having a silly name and a silly Glenn Miller swing ditty, "I've Got a Gal in Kalamazoo" to its credit. Kalamazoo means "boiling pot" to the indigenous Potawatomi Indians. It is a city dominated by the Upjohn Company, a pleasant American town that could be anywhere in the Midwest, like Garrison Keillor's Lake Wobegon, where all the folks are friendly and all the men have hair.

In the airport, there's still a volunteer handing out travel brochures about Kalamazoo at 11:30 P.M. My haired hotel clerk worries that I get a proper dinner after my midnight arrival. The waitress at Denny's is slow but polite. The haired cabbie gabs without being rude as he drives deftly over icy city streets.

A sweet, average place.

Like a Stephen King village in Maine.

Everything looks normal, even peaceful. But evil—*evil hair!*—bubbles just below the surface.

Hairy tommyknockers at my door. Beware the hairy tommyknockers. . . . Lead us not into minoxidil and deliver us from evil. . . .

In the morning, I step into the sixteen-degree freeze to meet two lieutenants of the Evil Empire that is Upjohn, the otherwise-benign multi-billion-dollar drugmaker behind minoxidil, the semioperable baldness potion marketed nationally as Rogaine. The original name, Regain, was viewed by the FDA as too optimistic and dropped.

"Goin' to the Taj Mahal?" my cabbie says with a chuckle. More like the Taj Mahair, I say to myself.

I will only have a few hours in the enemy camp. Only two interviews, one with a top marketing manager, Tim Thieme, the other with the director of the hair-growth research unit, Dr. Gerald Zins. No good reason was given for the refusal to let me see the labs where minoxidil is prepared. But I have infiltrated! I have gone where no baldness activist has gone before!

Nothing special about the Upjohn headquarters, save for the big Rogaine lobby display. The building (number eighty-eight) is heavily recessed from the main road, and is one of more than one hundred buildings Upjohn has occupied in Kalamazoo.

Better to hide the evil far from the populace.

The only animate objects without hair during my time in the Haired HQ were chrome domed robots delivering the day's mail. Several whirred quietly and efficiently through the wide mazelike corridors of the huge building, stopping at each office and refusing to commit the sins of human clerks: lallygagging and schmoozing. Robots are all business.

My guide, publicist Kaye Bennett, is lushly haired. She is a stouthearted minoxidilist, living and breathing the Gospel According to Rogaine. Her job is to defend minoxidil against all written and broadcast threats, foreign and domestic, and I have no doubt that she would lop off my shiny dome if I led a regiment of bald revolutionaries on an assault of building eighty-eight. But I will not reveal myself as Baldman here—if they discover me, I may have to enter the Unhaired Witness Protection Program and will probably have to wear a toupee—so Kaye's defenses are down. Her only job is to provide me with the material necessary to prove to me that minoxidil is the one, the only, the most effective, the *only* hair-growth drug okey-dokeyed by the United States Food and Drug Administration. She makes a friendly bet that I won't ask any questions of Thieme or Zins that she hasn't heard in the thousand press interviews she's fielded since the FDA approval came in the summer of 1988. I assure her I will win the wager. But her look tells me, No, she's heard it all.

Thieme is an overhaired thirtyish yuppie who sits very primly, hands clasped together for our hour together. His blue suit is neat. So is his dark, parted hair. You could tell he grew up happily as the boy next door to the family with the hairy tommyknockers. He'll never lose his mane, which was probably on his resume when he applied to market Rogaine. It was clear what he thought of bald activists like me.

"The 'bald-is-beautiful' people are a wing way out here," he says, gesturing to a far area on the right edge of his desk, "a very small minority." Who *is* this guy, the Spiro Agnew of hair growth, prattling like a hirsute kneejerk reactionary about the nattering nabobs of baldism? How dare he place people like me and the sagacious bald deity John Capps, head of the Bald-Headed Men of America, way out on the far right wing and place the unhaired masses, most of the 30 million bald men in America, who Thieme says "panic about losing their hair," in the mainstream?

But if there are so many of us panicky bald men, why haven't we crashed down the doors of pharmacies across the country? Here is a pseudo–miracle drug whose sales, Upjohn's protests aside, are disappointing. If only 10 percent of America's bald bought minoxidil, at about $700 a year, it should be a $2.1 billion drug. It won't be. It won't *ever* be. Analysts estimate that it may peak between $100 million and $200 million. There are several wonderful reasons for the basic failure of Rogaine, problems that would not bedevil it if it worked better.

- It's expensive, about sixty dollars a month, putting it up in the *very* pricey level of prescription drugs.

- It's not for a sickness. For high blood pressure or extreme pain you'll pay plenty to ease your woes. For falling hair, people are not so willing.
- It's not something doctors will readily prescribe, because *they* don't perceive the need. Doctors don't say, "Mr. Sandomir, your cholesterol is high. Your triglycerides are off the scale. And you're balder than anybody I've ever seen! So here's a prescription for Rogaine."
- It's not likely to work very well. Even Upjohn's own statistics bear this out: only 8 percent of the men in their tests showed dense regrowth while 31 percent reported moderate growth. Other tests reported even worse results, and dermatologists writing in a British medical journal said Rogaine is useless for 90 percent of all men. If your Darvon or Tylenol or tetracycline worked 10 to 40 percent of the time, you would not be satisfied.
- Its TV advertising stinks. Even Upjohn's folks come close to admitting that. You've seen the ads. There's the shot of the silent Man on the Beach, during which the screen only advises that, "If you're concerned about hair loss . . . see your doctor." There's the curly-blond Man in the Mirror, with barely any hair loss, who says, "I'm not bad now. But I wouldn't mind looking better" (blatant antibaldness discrimination there). There's a third from a dermatologist that ends with a message asking viewers to call an Upjohn number.

Why such bad advertising? It's not entirely Upjohn's fault. If Upjohn wanted to use the name Rogaine in the spots, it would have to name all the medical and side-effect information about it, an FDA requirement that would produce a very long, very

Be Brave...
Be Bold...
Be Bald!

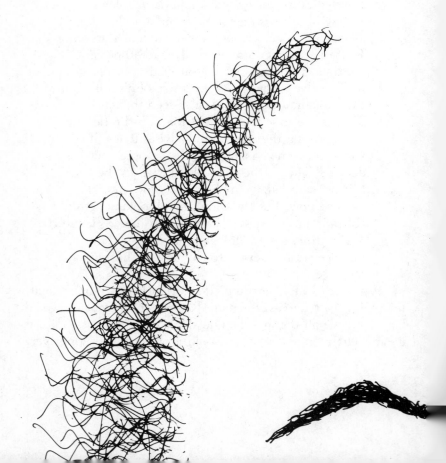

For maximum effect,
place book against your head
and view in a mirror.

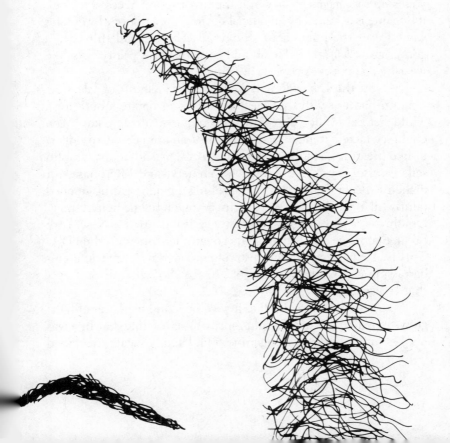

boring commercial. In newspaper and magazine ads, none of them zippity-doo-dah, Upjohn prints all the Rogaine data it can't fit on TV.

So, here's a product that is inadequately promoted, doesn't work well, isn't readily prescribed, is unnecessary and is overpriced. No wonder that in the Evil Empire, the overhaired executive suite is losing hair over minoxidil, the most overhyped, underused drug in America today.

"Like everybody, we thought this would be a huge market," said Thieme. "It's still a big market, but not as big as we thought five years ago."

The purchase of Rogaine by a balding man has to rank with condoms and tampons on the Red-Faced Scale. They're all embarrassing to buy—an admission that you or someone close to you is up to *something!*—even if the first two *are* necessary. Even if Rogaine is acquired by an official doctor's prescription, I wouldn't want to set the pharmacist thinking, "This cueball thinks he's gonna grow *hair?* Ha! He should read the fine print!" It's like wearing a toupee—people will *know!*

So you think *buying* it is embarrassing? Think of *selling* it. Upjohn had to swish that idea around its corporate mouth for a while before swallowing hard and saying meekly, Okay. You could see its reluctance. First, Rogaine is an unnecessary product, unlike the drugs Upjohn makes to work on *real* ailments; Upjohn sells *necessary* stuff like Xanax, for anxiety, and Micronase, for diabetes. Second, the thought of selling a baldness drug smelled faintly like hawking snake oil in a traveling medicine show. Upjohn is a century-old company, is listed on the New York Stock Exchange and is tied to the government through the FDA. This is, Rogaine aside, an upstanding company. Anything embarrassing can really hurt the old image. So why sell that . . . that . . . *hair stuff?*

"Upjohn didn't see itself as a developer and marketer of hair-growth medicine," says Gerald Zins, whose receding hairline was not led into fullness by using minoxidil. "This concept incubated

around here for a long time before it developed a level of ac-
ceptability. The connotation of hair growth was a matter of
concern to some individuals. That kind of research took some
getting used to."

Zins isn't neat. He's got a bit of the rumpled scientist about
him. His office in a former hospital a few miles away from the
Haired HQ is a mess of boxes and documents. He's been at
Upjohn through all its minoxidil testing, since the days when
minoxidil was a blood-pressure drug and scientists accidentally
discovered that it grew hair on patients.

Even Zins admits that the chief problem with it is it doesn't
work too well for growing hair, though it makes a helluva good
drug to lower your hypertension. His hair-growth research unit
is working on improving it and even creating an entirely new
drug. But so far, no luck. It's frustrating, maybe enough to tear
his hair out. They don't know if anything they come up with
will help more than a small minority of baldies.

Halfway through my talk with Zins, I win my bet with Kaye
Bennett, and in the process, emerge with damning information.
I ask Zins about the animals his unit used to test how well
minoxidil worked. Mice and rats, the usual suspects. Then comes
the magic words: "Stumptailed macaque monkeys." Why pick
on these primates, these aggressive, screechy evolutionary cous-
ins to man? Well, virtually all the little macaques (guys and gals)
go bald in a process eerily similar to male-pattern baldness. But
it's a little different with them: their hairline starts just above
their eyebrows, so at puberty, about age four, their hair recedes
back to where our hairlines generally begin, and the loss often
appears in a triangular pattern. The rest of the macaques' bodies
remain shaggy-haired, which reminds me of me: I'm bald on top
and inordinately overhaired on my back and chest. Maybe we're
closer in evolution than anyone originally thought.

These macaques are my people!!!

Now comes the question that wins my bet with Kaye Bennett.

"Do the still-haired macaques make fun of the bald ones?"

I ask. It's a reasonable question. Monkeys chatter, squawk and point a lot, behavior that could add up to antibaldness prejudice. Not a chance, though. I should have known that the macaques were better adjusted than humans.

"No," Zins says, a smile altering his dour demeanor. "That's not their basis for establishing a pecking order."

Not the way it is with humans, he might have added.

My first thoughts about the bald monkeys turn silly, to casting a macaque couple in a Rogaine commercial. As they walk down a beach, the neurotic male, who has the minuscule self-confidence of comedian Richard Lewis, says, "Honey, did you see how big my bald spot got? Should I call the vet for some minoxidil? Do I still look cute? I don't look bad now, but I'd like to look better."

The Minoxidil Macaques live one or two to a cage (squeeze cages that immobilize them for easier testing) at a primate center in Madison, Wisconsin, where they were born and bred to lend their balding pates to Upjohn. Although stumptailed macaques are a threatened species, one step below endangered, tests can be performed on them if they are born in captivity or were shipped here before the end of 1977.

In Madison, each day for several years, the macaques had their little heads brushed with minoxidil (and the joke's on Upjohn, because the goop worked better on the monkeys than it does on men). These are, by some accounts, aggressive, ornery monkeys, so it was only by caging them into obedience that they could be made to submit to minoxidil testing.

I ask Jerry Stone, the mammal curator at the Gladys Porter Zoo in Brownsville, Texas, what his pair of aging macaques, Pops and Pancho, would do if he invaded their primate island—where the little devils like to steal meat from the much larger gorillas—armed with a brush and a bottle filled with minoxidil. "They'd be off the walls," he says. "It would be a traumatic experience for them."

So who are the figurative monkeys here? After millions of

years of evolution, members of our higher species are reduced to spending years rubbing minoxidil on the receding hairlines of monkeys. It's food—or hair—for thought.

A journal article about the minoxidil testing of the monkeys shows photographs of the sad-eyed macaques during four stages of experimentation. I thought about how well the shots would look in an ad for the Hair Club for Macaques. The slogan? "I'm Not Only a Monkey—I'm a Client."

I am not sure if I understand the haired evil around me any more now than before I established my beachhead in Kalamazoo. I'm sure *they* think they're doing necessary work. And I'm equally sure that the few men who swear by what Rogaine has wrought on their heads see no evil. And I'm certain that I'll be visiting stumptailed macaques as soon as possible to kiss them on their bare foreheads.

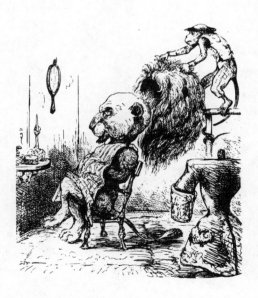

But I am also certain that Upjohn's aim is more demonic than the toupeemeisters' or the weavers' or transplanters'. No other antibald entity has spent as much money as Upjohn to create and promote a product that would prove to the bald that there is something wrong with them if they believe that bald is perfectly satisfying. *You don't look bad now, but you could look better! Hair is better than skin!* They've tried to capitalize on the ancient desire for a miracle cure and the modern hope for a magic bullet. That so many bald men have withstood Upjohn's assault is testimony to their strong resistance to being one of the suckers Upjohn hoped would be born every minute.

Through its sponsorship, Upjohn may enslave monkeys to test the stuff, but they can't imprison the so-called right-wing Bald Is Beautiful fringe. It is the banality of the well-meaning, good-citizen Upjohn that incorrectly *assumes* that tens of millions of men would storm their pharmacies for their monthly fix of the semioperable Rogaine that is at the heart of the Evil Empire of Upjohn.

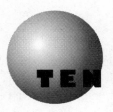

RUNNING FROM BALDNESS, OR, WOULD YOU RUB DOG URINE, BAT MILK OR HIPPO FAT ON YOUR HEAD?

○

IT ISN'T JUST the modern-day, media-fomented obsession with our looks that has sent unhaired folk looking for the latest baldness cure. From ancient days, there has been abundant evidence of freakish concoctions brewed to "cure" the terribly deadly scourge of baldness. Sad thing is, most of them sound as if they came from Grandpa Munster's book of potions and are as plausible as starting a brew with "eye of newt" down in the family dungeon.

Of all the potions that have come to the attention of my pate (and the one Grandpa Munster, that well-known vampire bat, would most relate to) none is odder than bat milk—or, musically (you know the words, *Batman* fans!), Da-da-da-da-da-da-da-da-da-da-da-da-da-da-da-da-da BAT MILK! BAT MILK! BAT MILK! Yes, bat milk, strange suckling source of batlet nourishment doubling as a better baldness brew than FDA-approved minoxidil—if you believe Swiss farmer Gerhardt Flit and the *Sun*, a supermarket tabloid where I found this, ahem, authoritative account.

On a fine Swiss spring morning, Farmer Flit was alone in his barn, a circumstance that was always dangerous for the eminent bat-agronomist. A few bats hung in the rafters. Seems then that a mommy bat in Farmer Flit's barn dripped some milk on his head. As he recalled: "I wiped it off. I thought it was a bat dropping but I looked in my hand and saw it was white. The next morning I woke up with hairs sprouting out of my head and the palm of my hand."

This moment, of course, is the Swiss equivalent of Alexander Graham Bell's "Come here, Watson, I need you."

Far from fretting, Farmer Flit tested his hypothesis. He snatched a mommy bat from her nest and squeezed her tiny udder, rendering forth a few drops of milk. Farmer Flit wasted no time in applying it to his head. Hairs, he said, quickly grew "like wild weeds." Though Farmer Flit apparently continued to engage in bat squeezing, he altered his tactic to rubbing an entire mommy bat on his head when he desired treatment. The treatment bore fruit of a kind: within six weeks, Farmer Flit had a lot of Bat Hair.

And so, Farmer Flit, a resident of a country that, if it were not neutral, would surely see to it that its people would have something better to do than squeeze milk out of bats, attracted hundreds of bats to his bat barn, and created a colony of sixty nursing mommy bats. He feeds them high-grade moths, then milks them with a mini–cow milker, yielding milk that he bottles and sells for $3,500 an ounce. "It's a lot of money," Farmer Flit admits, "but it's easier than rubbing a screeching bat across your head."

Farmer Flit is part of a long, dishonorable and silly tradition. Thanks in part to Roy Blount's book *It Grows on You*, here is a roster of the most bizarre baldness potions you're liable to see anywhere!

1. Dog urine (head firmly placed under dog's haunches).
2. Equal parts Abyssinian greyhound's heel, date blossoms and asses' hooves. Boil in oil.
3. Onion juice.
4. Bear grease and laudanum.
5. Almond oil, ammonia, Spanish fly and lemon oil.
6. Equal parts fat of a lion, hippo, crocodile, goose, snake and ibex (yielding the Wild Kingdom Coif).

7. Spider webs. (Charlotte had hair, why not you?)
8. Coconut fat, sulphur oil and mustard oil.
9. Three parts Peruvian balsam, 3 parts castor oil, 35 parts alcohol, 4 parts Spanish fly, 40 parts rosewater. (Almost guaranteed to make you look like Julio Iglesias.)
10. Pigeon dung and honey simmered over a slow fire.
11. Jerusalem artichoke juice (*only* from Jerusalem).
12. Dew from St. John's wort. (That's *wort*, not wart, though a wart would do you as much good.)
13. Estrogen cream (so you'll enjoy being a girl).
14. Dates, dogs' paws, asses' hooves ground up and cooked in oil and rubbed vigorously into head.
15. Cleopatra's remedy: burned domestic mice, horse teeth, bear grease and deer marrow (but it didn't work for Big Julie Caesar, and Mark Antony didn't need it).
16. Hedge garlic.
17. Ground donkey teeth boiled in oil (which will make you feel like an ass).
18. Various combinations of myrtle leaves, pine tree bark, white wine, oil of radish seed, sorrel, myrrh, willow leaves, oil of green juniper berries, wormwood, fern roots, linseed oil, bruised almonds, wheat bran and mastic powder.
19. Horse saliva. (Well, have you ever seen a bald horse?)
20. Cow-licking (resulting in the cowlick, grown first from the heretofore unknown bald spot on the top of Little Rascal Alfalfa's head).

There is plenty of pseudo-hairism afoot around the world (and here I cite the work of dermatologist Albert Kligman), some of it pure humbuggery, some of it making a bizarre form of sense (even if the method doesn't really work).

Oh, those wacky Egyptians. Not only did they, according to the ancient historian Herodotus, have a professional called a "physician of the head," but they had some unusual ideas about how to cure baldness. According to one of their ancient papyri, the Egyptians engaged exorcists, said Kligman, to invoke the "eternal immobile Aton—a disk or sun—to fight the malefic divinity that mastered the summit of the bald head." That makes it sound as if Edmund Hillary had scaled the summit of Mount Baldy and rubbed off all the hair with his mountaineering boots.

The Japanese are no less strange. They are obsessed with keeping their hair. Failing that, they jump quickly to buy toupees or just about anything that promises a return to hairs past. One popular pseudo-remedy is a brush that buyers are told must be struck upon their head two hundred times, twice daily.

(*Beat me with your rhythm stick! Beat me! Beat me!*)

The brush keeps track of the number of strikes so the user doesn't lose count while he's bludgeoning himself. The trauma may increase blood flow, but probably isn't the best thing to do psychologically. Kligman reports that the brush is marketed with this encouraging slogan: "Japanese men are beaten at work, they are beaten at home, and beating makes strong men!" Some marketing campaign.

In France, rum alcohol, beef marrow and bergamot oil is recommended, or an extract of fresh bovine (that's cow or bull to you and me) heart and lecithins. In Hungary, it's horseradish, mustard oil, orange and lemon peels and egg yolk. In the U.S.S.R., it's acupuncture.

Kligman is a dermatologist with a sense of humor. He notes that scientists know that certain painful treatments create inflammations that stimulate hair growth. There's the case of the mentally retarded patient who gnawed on one part of his forearm. Hairs grew. You can grow hair by rubbing lesions. Ancient icemen, who kept hitting their heads with blocks of ice, were known to grow hair. Yet, says yukster-dermatologist Kligman, "Physical trauma to the scalp is hardly a feasible treatment."

One of the foremost students of pseudo–baldness cures was one Lucy Ricardo, redhead extraordinaire and wife to Ricky, who, in one episode of *I Love Lucy*, was worried that Ricky's hair was departing. It wasn't, but he deeply feared looking like his best friend, the aggressively bald Fred Mertz. Lucy, failing to convince Ricky that his hair was intact, embarked on a campaign to concoct a treatment so miserable that Ricky would give up, and, if need be, accept the Fate of Fred, which never came. (To the day he died, Desi Arnaz had nearly all his Cuban hair.) So, after visiting a hair alchemist (a ghoulish, toupeed vulture hawking creams, ointments, tonics, scrapers, dilators, suction devices and agitators), and inviting a depressing group of bald men over to her apartment for comparison with Ricky's bulky head protein, Lucy invented the Lucy Ricardo Torture System of Hair Restoring, which bears a rather close resemblance to a number of "cures," past and present.

"Your roots won't know what hit them," Lucy promises as she begins the treatment. First came the hand-held vibrator, which jiggled Ricky's head like those toy Bobble Heads with baseball caps on them, and, "made my head feel like it's on fire" (a sure portent of future hair growth). Next came Lucy's presentation of a stocking, which she had Ricky wear overnight on his

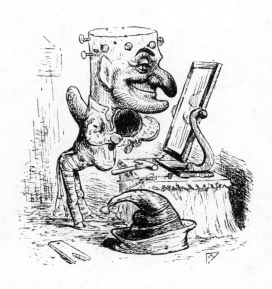

head to cover the mustard plaster she applied to his head. The following step had Lucy applying oil, vinegar and eggs to Ricky's head. "Why don't you put in some anchovies and make a Caesar salad?" asks an incredulous and gooey Ricky.

Was it any worse than pigeon dung or burned mice?

For the final sad word on the psychology of hair replacement "cures," we must now turn to the sagacious Mr. Mertz. "Nothing has ever been invented," says Fred, "that a man won't try if he thinks he can get his hair back."

So true, so true.

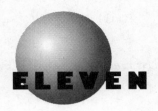

ELEVEN

BALDLETT'S QUOTATIONS

○

Fred Astaire's got no hair.
Nor does a chair.
Or a chocolate eclair.
And where is there hair on a pear?
Nowhere, mon frère.
—GEORGE CARLIN

"Cure baldness." Those ads always bug me. It's not like
athlete's foot or a headache; take two aspirin and it's gone
by morning. What is there to cure? It's not contagious.
Jonas Salk didn't spend any time trying to isolate baldness.
—JOE GARAGIOLA

Go up, baldhead; go up, baldhead.
—2 KINGS 2:23

(One assumes this means that the bald will reach
heaven first.)

A man of my limited resources cannot presume to have a
hairstyle. Get on and cut it.
—WINSTON CHURCHILL, to a barber

(I'll bet he never spent sixty-five dollars on a stylist
who specializes in bald heads!)

*On all their heads shall be baldness and every beard
cut off.*
—ISAIAH 15:2

(A perfect world.)

You make your kind of money, you don't lose your hair.
—JONATHAN WINTERS, to
Johnny Carson

(It's true. Talk show hosts tend to keep their hair.
Look at Steve Allen, Pat Sajak, Phil Donahue, Oprah
Winfrey, Merv Griffin, Mike Douglas.)

*There's not time for a man to recover his hair that grows
bald by nature.*
—WILLIAM SHAKESPEARE

(Baldness is forever; a toupee only masks it.)

*Adlai, get rid of the fringes. Erase the dividing line. Then
no one will know whether you are a genuine egghead or
not. Besides, completely bald men are more sensual.*
—YUL BRYNNER'S advice to
presidential candidate Adlai Stevenson

(Yul was not only a fine actor, but also a
philosopher-king.)

*Does not the very nature of things teach you that if a man
has long hair, it is a disgrace to him?*
—SAINT PAUL

(Thus, the highest form of human respect is baldness.)

*I can't verify that bald men are better lovers. But my
hunch is that a man who has lost his hair—or is losing it*

fast and isn't preoccupied by the fact—is generally superior in bed.
—Letter writer to DEAR ABBY

(I agree.)

Fellas, there she is. There's the little lady who put us out of business.
—CARL REINER as Alan Brady in *The
Dick Van Dyke Show,* talking to his
toupees after his baldness was revealed
by Laura Petrie (Mary Tyler Moore)

Interview magazine: *What would you do if you went bald?*

Brian Bosworth: *It would suck. It would really suck.*

(What self-respecting human would cut his hair like
the Boz's?)

*Burt Reynolds needs to emancipate his hairpieces . . . and
bare his scalp to the wind. But would that work? There's
no reason to believe that stripped of his Velcro curls
Reynolds would be transformed into a sullen hard-on like
Robert Duvall or a salted egg like Sean Connery.*
—JAMES WOLCOTT in *Vanity Fair*

(Please, Burt, please. Show us your scalp! Do it for
Loni.)

I'm not bald. I'm having my hair surgically removed.
—comedian BILL MASTERS

(And mine just shrank in the washing machine.)

*While television news tolerates degrees of baldness, it
seldom accepts both baldness and glasses. Middle America:*

Where else would a balding guy in glasses hang out?
　—New York Times *critic* JOHN CORRY
on CBS Morning Show *host Harry*
Smith

(A bald guy with glasses hangs out in my apartment.
Me.)

Skin is definitely in and who in the world wants to look
like Phil Donahue or Boy George?
　—HAROLD FLEISCHMAN, *voted*
"Smoothest Head in America"
for 1988

I'd tear the hair out of my head, but I don't have any.
　—Chicago Cubs *manager* DON ZIMMER
in a frustrating moment

(I know the feeling, Don, I know the feeling.)

You fob us off with fictitious hair—your dirty bald scalp is
covered with locks represented in paint. You have no
occasion for a barber for your head; you may shave
yourself much better, Phoebus, with a sponge.
　—Roman *epigrammist* MARTIAL *on*
the strange first-century practice of
painting hair on bald scalps

By the time he was manager of Archie Moore, Jack
Kearns [Jack Dempsey's manager] had grown a head full of
skin but when he was a young man weighing gold dust in a
government assay house, he had abundant black hair.
　—RED SMITH

(This from a man who first lost any hint of red, and
then lost his hair.)

When our crew from ESPN walks into the Duke Indoor
Stadium down in Durham before a game, they have a
standard chant. Half the crowd yells "Bald," the other
yells, "Head." And then alternately, "Bald!" "Head!"
"Bald!" "Head!" And they're pointing at me and
stomping and everything. Of course, I play it up. I go get
a towel from the manager and start shining my dome and
the crowd goes absolutely bananas.
    —DICK VITALE, ESPN college
        basketball commentator

(A well-adjusted man after my own pate.)

Covering his sensual dome [with a wig] is like putting
clothes on Lady Godiva.
    —MARLENE DIETRICH, on Yul Brynner

(And this woman knew bald beauty when she saw it.)

I call it the Watergate. I cover up everything I can.
    —former baseball player JOE TORRE
        describes his combover coif

Nobody's ever happy with what they have. People with
curly hair want straight and people with straight want curly
and bald people want everyone to be blind.
    —comedian RITA RUDNER

(Not entirely true. We just want every overhaired
    person to be bald for a day or two.)

How could I hide it? It's gone. It's outta here. My advice
is just go with it. To me, people who wear hairpieces look
so dumb. So bad, so dumb, much dumber than the guy
without hair. I can understand it for an actor. He's got a
certain image to maintain. But it's weird to see just regular

*people walking around with hairpieces on. That's what's so
hip to me about a guy like Sean Connery. The guy is
unbelievably handsome; he's a sexy guy. He says, "Screw
it, man, this is what I look like," and women don't think
any less of him; they probably like him more.*
—ROB REINER in US magazine

(The Meathead turns bald activist.)

We don't have time for rugs, plugs or drugs.
—JOHN CAPPS, head head of the Bald-
Headed Men of America

(My hero.)

*The truest metaphor for the man is his hair. Here is a
grown man, happily married, who for reasons of vanity or
political calculation chooses to wear his hair as if it were a
rug. Not even a good rug, but something that looks like it's
chopped out of a YMCA carpet. . . . For what reason?
We don't know. After all, what is wrong with being a
nice, normal balding person like Jack Nicholson or George
Washington? Why try to make those lonesome follicles look
more dense? Why glue these strands together so they look
like a vegetable burger? . . . The sprayed and coddled hair
still lies on his skull like a fur-bearing yarmulke.*
—*New York Post* columnist PETE
HAMILL on defeated New York mayoral
candidate Rudolph Giuliani's
combover

*Who would have supposed that this grotesque ornament, fit
only for an African chief, would be considered
indispensably necessary for the administration of justice in
the middle of the nineteenth century.*
—British author JOHN CAMPBELL on
the already-outmoded practice of
barristers and judges wearing wigs
in court

*One of us besides Gracie had been wearing a toupee since
that person was twenty-seven or twenty-eight years old,
and the other person had never said a word about it. I
would have my toupee made to look exactly like my hair
had looked, too, but who could remember what it had
looked like? At night, I'd put my toupee on a dummy
head, and Gracie would put one of her wigs on a dummy
head, and the two heads would be right next to each other
on the bureau. I got a strange feeling when I looked at
them; I felt like I was sitting behind ourselves in
the theater.*
—GEORGE BURNS, on his career-long
addiction to hairpieces

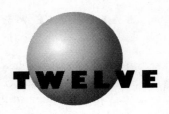

TWELVE

THE BALD OF RIGHTS: A REAL THOUSAND POINTS OF LIGHT

○

EVERY DAY, A new group wants to be recognized and granted the civil rights due them. Gays, the unborn, women, the disabled, Vietnam veterans, blacks, Hispanics, fat folks, poor folks, American flag–burners. I even heard about a dwarf named Little T who, on the wrong side of right on *Donahue*, seemed to need a code of rights to continue to volunteer himself as a paid projectile for beer-bellied barflies to hurl in the air in the bizarre pseudo-sport called dwarf-tossing. If Little T wants rights, give them to him. Let Congress pass the Dwarf-Tossing Rights Act of 1990. If LBJ were still president, he'd do it. He wanted justice for all.

Plenty of people need legal rights to pursue their goals and for protection from those who would infringe upon their freedoms. That's what the Bill of Rights is about. Same for the Bald of Rights.

We of the unhaired persuasion must be allowed to pursue our life without sneers and derision from hairists, hair stylists and hair replacers. We want people to look into our eyes when we converse, not onto our head.

We are equal under the law with haired folk and we should be treated as such. But we are not and we know it.

It is time we rise up now or be crucified upon a cross of hair. We are not asking for special treatment or special protection, just a very simple Bald of Rights that lets us start at the same place as the hairy guys. Think of it as affirmative action for the bald class. The 30 million bald men in the United States cross every ethnic, racial, religious and sexual line.

We are the true Majority Minority. But until now we've been a Silent Baldority. That must change.

I tried to make this point in a letter to President Bush. It is a tactic I readily admit stealing from Garrison Keillor in his plea to President Carter for shy rights. Keillor wrote the letter, but he was too shy to send it. I'm not shy, so here's the letter I sent to our haired president on October 2, 1989.

Dear Mr. President,

I must commend you on the calm, intelligent and reasoned tone you've brought to the White House. I didn't vote for you, but I'm starting to wonder why I didn't. You, the First Lady and the First Kids are an exemplary family to lead us into the 1990s.

But I must be critical in one area. So far, I've heard nothing from you or your administration about the rights of the bald. Sir, I know it sounds silly in light of your feelings and pronouncements about the rights of the unborn and the rights of other constituencies aggrieved in some manner. But the need for a codified set of rights for the unhaired remains an unaddressed issue that may dog your presidency.

I know you may not have heard much about the need for bald rights. You and your sons are filled with hair, so your attention has not focused on this serious problem. It's my feeling, incidentally, that most politicians who aspire to the presidency have an abundance of hair. (My scalp doctor says it has to do with an overabundance of active hormones.) Just look at the field of Democrats and Republicans who vied for the 1988 presidential nominations: all but one, Joe Biden, had masses of hair, a pretty mean feat for a bunch of men between forty and seventy.

Although you are to be commended for your appointments of Dick Cheney and Marlin Fitzwater, two fine bald public servants, you have yet to address Bald Rights.

You may ask me, Why Bald Rights? Good question.

We need a Bill of Bald Rights to keep people from asking, "Did you know you were losing hair?" or "Have you ever thought of wearing a toupee?" or "Aren't you a little young to be going bald?"

We need Bald Rights to ban advertisements for hair replacements that promise to "cure" something that isn't a sickness. We need Bald Rights to eliminate the prejudice that comes from being pointed out in a crowded room as "that bald guy in the corner." Would they point out a different man as "that haired guy in the corner?" We need Bald Rights to eliminate toupees.

We need Bald Rights to stamp out baldness-driven housing discrimination ("I'm sorry," one landlord told a friend, "we were hoping for someone with hair") and job bias ("We were hoping for someone more dynamic, someone with, say, some hair on that head," a potential employer once told the head of the Bald-Headed Men of America). We need Bald Rights to push Congress to enact legislation that will allow us to redress our baldness discrimination grievances in federal court.

Mr. President, only you can address this burning issue. Thirty million bald men await your answer.

Sincerely,
Richard Sandomir

The president has not responded yet. But I know he will. After all, to whom do you think he was referring when he talked about the "thousand points of light"? Haired heads don't shine. But he knows we baldies shine an eternal light into the future.

PREAMBLE: We the bald people of the world, in order to form a more perfect personal Dome, to establish justice and tonsorial tranquility, and provide for the defense of our naked heads, do ordain and establish the Bald of Rights.

Article I. By executive order, all written or verbal claims, either implicit or explicit, that baldness is a curable disease shall be banned from public discourse. There's nothing wrong with you when you don't have hair. You don't have to wear hairpieces. When you're bald, you don't have a trace of fever, bacteria, or viral infection. You don't get the shakes and you actually lose a few ounces off the top. Thinking of baldness as a curable disease conjures up images of a Code Hair emergency in the Hairmeister Hospital. A hysterical bald man is brought in by ambulance, strapped down to a stretcher. "Calling Dr. Sperling, patient in emergency, suffering from acute baldness. Needs emergency weave. Patient in follicle arrest."

Article II. No bald person shall feel compelled to wear a hairpiece. Even when you're adorned with the best of them, someone will know about it. Everybody you knew before you plunked the alien hair onto your head will know you're wearing

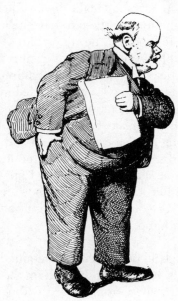

it. When you least expect it—in a hurricane, in a stiff gale or while swimming in the pool—your piece may part company with your head. Even if it never does—do you want to suffer from the paranoid thought that it might? Think of this charitably: the hair you wear comes from poor Italian and Asian women who shear themselves for your vanity. Expect to see commercials for needy women with buns atop their head, pleading for your nickels and dimes to help *them* get a wig to cover up the gap left when they clipped for your sake. Show compassion. Let them keep their hair.

Article III. No bald man shall have to endure people staring at his head during conversations. The bald shall have the right to stare at the sexual organs or mammary glands of the head-starers and shall not be prosecuted for the embarrassment this may cause others.

Article IV. Congress shall make no laws quartering bald men against their will and forcing them to have hair transplants upon their scalps. They're bloody. They're painful. They don't always work. You'll look like somebody just ran over your head with a tractor. Think of the procedure: healthy hair plugs from the back of your head are forcibly removed and injected into holes punched in the front of your head. Transplanters do this with sharp hole punchers usually used to make cancer biopsies. Then, when they don't work, you might have to do it again and again. Assuming the transplant works, realize it will take months before it looks like anything but aerial photographs of Kansas corn. Until it grows in, you'll either look stupid (and boy are people going to talk to your head) or you'll have to wear a hat for three or four years like Roy Clark did.

Article V. No bald person shall be required to use minoxidil for the rest of his life. Depending upon the study you read, minoxidil works anywhere from never to 30 percent of the time in growing some babylike, fuzzy hair in areas of almost negligible hair loss. The newly grown hair won't mix in well with the hair around it. They won't get along. You have to apply it every day for the rest of your life. If you stop using it, any new hair will fall out.

Article VI. Congress shall enact laws that prohibit the growth of hair very long on one side of a man's head for the purpose of swinging it over to the other side to create a false sense of hair, or "combover." This right not to look ridiculous is done in the interest of the public aesthetic and for the comboverist's good, for combing over a bald spot is even more transparent than wearing a hairpiece.

Article VII. The legislative branch shall ensure that no bald man need worry about what a woman thinks of an unhaired head. They really don't care. Forget the surveys you may have read about; they're paid for by hairmeisters. Any antibald sentiment on the part of women is purely a first-impression across-the-room response. Most guys think women care, but they really don't. If baldness detracts from a man's appeal, why did Yul Brynner and Telly Savalas become sex symbols only after shaving their heads? If you're covering up only because of a woman, remember this: the Fake Hair Police are always on the prowl— and women are absolutely spectacular at spotting a rug.

Article VIII. Bald men shall have the right, without fear of penalties, to hate men aged fifty years or more with too much hair. Such loathing shall be increased by a factor of 25 percent if the old fart's hair color is still his original. The list shall include Ronald Reagan, George Steinbrenner, Leonard Bernstein, Roger Moore, Michael Dukakis, Robert Wagner, Dan Rather, Joe DiMaggio, Senator Robert Dole, Sparky Anderson, Bill Cosby,

Walter Cronkite, Ed McMahon and any other old-timer you can name.

Article IX. Newspapers, magazines and other media shall be required to eliminate all use of the word *bald* as a description for a man in the following instances: (a) when a picture of the person accompanies the article and (b) as long as other men are not described as "haired." Journalistic rules, properly enforced, should require descriptions that emphasize the unusual and outstanding in a person. Baldness, however, is a description appropriate for 30 million men.

Article X. All heads, henceforth, shall be recognized as perfectly shaped for baldness. Misconceptions abound that only the right round head is well-suited for baldness, making some owners of ovoid, squarish and elliptical bald heads self-conscious and prone to purchases of hair replacements.

Article XI. The Civil Rights Act of 1964 shall be amended to include bald men among those who shall be free from employment and housing discrimination. Any breach that would result in denying a bald man the housing or job he desires because of the state of his head shall entitle him to the same rights and redress as other groups, plus treble monetary damages.

Article XII. In all situations tonsorial, the bald man shall enjoy the right to a speedy and discount haircut by a barber or stylist, rather than enduring a deliberately slow snipping designed to have the practitioner spend as much time on cutting the sides as he would spend on a fully haired customer.

Is this too much to ask? I think not. These should be the inalienable rights of all bald men, great and small. Write your congressman! Write the president, haired though he may be!

We must educate our underprivileged haired brethren, who know not what they do when they utter an antibald word or perform an antibald act. Only through enactment and enforcement of the Bald of Rights can this education be achieved.

If not now, when?

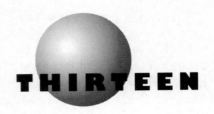

THIRTEEN

BLOOD, SWEAT AND PLUGS: THE TRUE UNTOLD STORY OF RESODDING YOUR HEAD SURGICALLY

○

ANYBODY WITH ANY restaurant savvy knows that no matter how good your duck à l'orange is, it's best not to head back into the kitchen to give your kudos to the chef. You might see how the food was prepared. When I was a summer camp waiter, I watched the salad man mix cole slaw in a vat with his dirty, sweaty, hairy bare arm. I swore off cole slaw for years.

Anybody who wants a hair transplant is better off a patient than an observer. Even done well, a transplant is bloody ugly and bloody disgusting.

I know.

I watched.

The guy with the holes in his scalp felt nothing.

I threw up.

I will not cast aspersions here on the talents of Dr. Gary Hitzig, who is a very nice, generous and accommodating man. Hitzig is a thin forty-year-old surgeon with a thick New York accent, a one-time teenage baldie and toupee wearer whose current hairline was resurrected from not one but two transplants.

I like Hitzig even if I have the true soul of a bald man and he is technically an enemy of the people. He makes no wild claims. He comforts and teases patients and lets them watch TV with a remote-control device of their own as he plunges his needles and surgical punches into their scalps. He's done seventeen thousand transplants, enough men to fill up Madison Square Garden for a New York-Rangers game.

I met Gary ten days before at a seminar he sponsored, and felt comfortable enough to tell him about this book and my odyssey through the bald world. Come to Rockville Centre, he beckoned. Watch some transplants.

Patient Peter C. sits in an examining room. What's left of his hair is a wispy dirty-blond. Sprouts of unkempt strands dot his head. He had a transplant from another doctor that took badly. The plugs are visible. The hairs that grew out of the plugs splay upward like cattails.

He'd be better off bald. As would we all.

Hitzig's first task is a scalp reduction. Scary term, scalp reduction. Sounds like something the Apaches invented some time ago. The very idea of what transplant doctors do to your head embodies principles taken either from the Indian wars or the Three Stooges: punching holes in your head (Nyuk, nyuk, nyuk!), pulling out skin and follicles (Moe! Moe!), injecting them back in (Hey Moe, Hey Moe!) and cutting out pieces of your scalp (Nyuk, nyuk, nyuk).

One thing scalp reduction won't do is stretch your scalp so your nose winds up on top of your head—assuming that it is done right. The principle at work here is that the scalp is pliable and has a lot of extra skin it doesn't really need. If you cut out bald skin, you reduce the hairless tundra. More haired scalp remains and you don't need to inject plugs in the reduced quadrant. But until the transplanters hypothesized that they could cut out scalp, no one really thought it was anything that anyone this side of George Armstrong Custer would want.

This is what happened to Peter C. and me, but first—hide your scalp. Hide your women and children. This isn't going to be pretty.

Peter sits quietly watching a situation comedy, with heavily absorbent gauze wrapped around his head. Hitzig wraps a gas mask around Peter's face and pumps nitrous oxide up his nose. Peter gets high. Then with a very long needle filled with heated xylocaine, Peter's scalp is numbed twenty separate times. Every plunge of the needle causes the scalp to puff up—the way it's supposed to, Hitzig explains. Trickles of blood go down Peter's head and into the gauze.

Each injection—and the puffing of the scalp—weakens my knees.

Meanwhile, Hitzig is talking nonstop.

Injection.

"Feeling all right?" Hitzig asks.

"Yep," says Peter.

Two seconds go by.

Injection.

"Feeling all right?"

"Yep."

Two seconds go by.

Injection.

"Feeling all right?"

"Yep."

"That's all the pain you're going to feel," promises Hitzig. "Really dreadful, huh? Better than Dr. Jones [not his real name], right?"

"Yeah, I felt everything that time," he says.

Peter's previous transplant was done painfully, he says, by Manhattan physician Dr. Joe Jones.

"Can you believe it," says Hitzig. "Jones said Peter was a bleeder."

Incredible!

As for me, I'm not feeling so well. I'm lightheaded. I duck out of the room to sit in a bloodless supply room. A medical assistant serves me a soda. He turns on a fan. I'm faint.

I return in time to see Dr. Hitzig, scalpel in hand, slice

Peter's scalp along the dividing line in the rear of his head between the hairless dome and the haired fringe. Blood gurgles and flows. The assistant puts pressure on the bloody area to slow the flow and dabs the blood with gauze. Hitzig's lengthwise slice continues in a curve three inches long, then to a width of about one inch.

"You're having a reduction," says Hitzig. "Isn't it awful?"

"I hear it," says Peter, "but I don't feel it."

But I'm feeling every slice of the scalp massacre. It's like the feeling you get when a baseball player gets hit by a ball in his groin and he can't hold it in front of fifty thousand people. What empathy you feel!

The blood flows. Hitzig scissors the bald flap and the pink skin beneath the scalp is now naked to the air. The blood drips down. The assistant dabs away while Hitzig makes easy patter.

Hitzig picks up the ends of skin on either side of the abyss and stretches them to show me how pliable the skin is and how easy it will be to stitch both sides together.

"A lot of doctors won't stitch it up until after the transplant," he says. "I'm doing it now."

I've had it. Hitzig sees it in my eyes. He's stitching together the scalp with black surgical thread, and suggests the bathroom is the second door to the right. "It happens to some people," he says as I leave the room.

I arrive in time to throw up. I am sure this is a symbolic upchuck on behalf of millions of bald men everywhere. I'm convinced my brethren would be proud of me. If they could see what I've seen. I'm both bloodied *and* bowed, and I'm proud of it.

You want hair? Prepare to bleed for it.

Weak-kneed and white-faced, I return to the operating theater (actually about the size of a dentist's office; Hitzig's tools include a modified dentist's drill). I find Hitzig in midtransplant.

This is less bloody but no more attractive.

Hitzig has already started the hair harvest. Peter now has one hundred tiny holes punched in the front of his head, made under much the same principle you'd use to punch holes into paper for a looseleaf. Up top where his hairline used to be now resides a symmetrical pattern of hairless holes. Into them will go healthy plugs of hairy follicles.

This is Hitzig's description of the tool he uses to kidnap the plugs from the back of Peter's head: "This is my design. Most people buy a power tool, but it's too heavy. So I use a commercial engine with minimum torque and little vibration with a modified dental tool that hooks bits into it." Hmm—the Black & Decker Hair Transplanter!

Sounds like something you could pick up at a local hardware store. "Hi, Pat Summerall here for True Value. . . ."

Out come the plugs. Hitzig's tool cuts out circular spaces in the back of Peter's head. Bing! Bing! Bing! This is easy!

"Feeling all right?"

"Yep."

"I'm not hurting you?"

"Nope."

The cuts go deeply enough to get skin, tissue and follicle (you can see the little tiny shaved-down hairs if you look closely). As Hitzig punches out the plugs, his assistant places them on gauze atop Peter's head. A second assistant places them in the new holes in Peter's head. The plugs are wider than the holes so when they are pushed in, they pop, like corks. The principle is that they stay there. You hope.

With the plugs now in, Hitzig sutures up the area from whence the plugs came. The skin stretches to allow several mini-reductions. Now there won't be a vacant area in the back where hair won't grow. Hair that surrounds the sutured area will grow over the scar. Hitzig marvels at the pliability of the skin of the scalp. "This guy's got Playtex living skin," he jokes.

I ask Peter why he's doing this, for surely he will feel discomfort and pain when the painkillers wear off.

"The worst thing about being bald," says Peter, who sells ladies' clothing, "is seeing your friends who all have the same

hair they had when they were fourteen. You feel gypped. Or you
see a bum. You never see a bald bum. They don't even take care
of their hair. It's all greasy and matted. But at least they have
it."

I stay to watch Hitzig do a series of minireductions on a "plug
junkie." This guy, Barry, has already had a transplant, giving
him a head of wavy curls. But Barry constantly examines his
head for tiny, vacant areas, which he begs and cajoles (and pays)
Hitzig to plug up. "He has a full head of hair," says an exasperated
Hitzig, "but still he complains."

I leave Hitzig's office, still lightheaded and weak-kneed. I
now know I can never have a transplant.

I have seen it.

I have vomited.

I am not convinced.

I feel peculiarly exhilarated. The soul of this bald man has
triumphed over the plugs of a surgeon. The impulse to surgically
repair my bare scalp is gone. My position remains impregnable.
My skin remains untouched. Hairless, yes—but untouched.

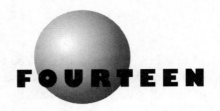

FOURTEEN

EXCLUSIVE INTERVIEW: I AM BALDMAN'S PATE!

○

PLEASE ENTER AND sign in please. Now tell us who you are.

I am his pate, the top of Richard Sandomir's head.

Tell us a little about your life, sir.

Oh, it's pretty simple. I walk around naked except for some hair on the sides and in the back.

You were once covered over, is that correct?

Are you kidding? Of course! Oy, a head of hair, like you shouldn't know from. It was one never-ending curl after another, so dense I thought I was in the middle of Sherwood Forest. I couldn't see a damned thing through it.

So you're happy the way you are?

Delirious. Wouldn't you be? I was buried for twenty years. When the hairs came off, I felt like Papillon swimming away from Devil's Island. When Dick—he hates to be called Dick, but I like teasing him—went to Spain, I saw Spain. A little hot, but nice. I wore a nice mesh cap that I saw through easily. When Dick saw the pope in Vatican City, I saw the pope. You should have seen the pope's pate. We had an instant rapport. I haven't been that happy since the day Dick was born.

How soon after Dick's birth did you go into the haired dungeon?

It happened real fast. Two, three months, tops. The curls grew like weeds. Dick's mom marveled at them, how they looked exactly like her mother's. If only she had left them alone.

What do you mean?

Well, when you're a pate, curls can sometimes be seen through.

184

You crane your neck a little, you can see through the ringlets. Thick, straight hair is murder, but if you get the right angle through curls, you can make out a building or a person. So what Dick's mom did was take him to the barber where this guy, who always smelled of Barbasol, would slick the curls down with some green goo. Closed up every view. I can live with an obstructed view. Always had, though this was worse than sitting in a bad seat at Fenway Park. But every time that green goop went on, I was dead meat. Sayonara to the world.

So you were closed off to the world for many years?

Yup. God knows, Dick didn't have a clue about what to do with his hair even when he stopped green-gooping me. From where I sat, he must have looked like a cross between Medusa and Don King. The curls were flying everywhere. He got Afro cuts, but in a week or two, it was out of control. He'd jab me with his damned Afro pick.

Let's get back to Dick going bald. When was that?

Let me see. I'd say he was about sixteen or seventeen when I saw some light at the end of the follicles. He didn't know he was balding until he was twenty or twenty-one.

Did you engineer the whole thing?

No, but I could have stopped it. It was so much fun I forgot.

But what could you have stopped?

Dick's got your basic male pattern baldness. That means his male hormones, his androgens, are running wild. It's not that he had too many or too few androgens. They were just out of control. I could have regulated it. I could have shut down the hormone spigot. But I figured, what the hell? Let's see what happens. And then, boy, the kicker came when his dihydrotestosterone went bananas. His hairs sucked up the stuff like a newborn to its mother's breast. The dihydro, as we pates call it, shrank his follicles, which made the hair grow shorter and shorter. After a while, it was rest in peace for those hairs. Of course, I could have slowed down the whole thing. But why? Pates have a one-track mind. We want to be naked. You know? Constantly.

But Dick was easy. Some pates never get to have as much fun as I have had in so short a time. Some of them wait forty, fifty or sixty years to see what I saw in less than ten. His hormones were flowing like Old Faithful.

Was there anything Dick could have done?

Not a thing.

Not even minoxidil?

This guy was too far gone for anything like that to work. By the time they came out with that stuff—and believe me, I'm glad I didn't have to have that goop put on me—Dick's follicles were so miniaturized and slow-growing that it would have been like planting corn seed in the Dust Bowl in the 1930s.

Do you see an irony in Dick's having so much body hair and nothing on top?

Not at all. Strip nine out of ten bald guys and you'll find unnatural growths of hair on their chests and backs. It's normal. See, while the old dihydro cuts off the hair supply up top, it

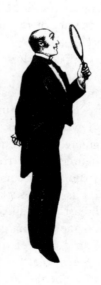

makes it run amuck everywhere else. Strange hormone, that dihydro. I'm surprised Dick doesn't carry a comb for his back. Jeez, have you seen the rug he's got back there? Enough hair for two toupees. Enough to cover an orangutan's back.

Why are you so hostile?

It's not hostility, pal, it's survival. It was bad enough that he had natural hair that blocked my view of the world. I got rid of that. And a wig would be worse. First, I'd have to try to see through the foundation that they stitch the hair into. Second, God forbid he buys a wig with artificial hair. It'd be like trying to see through Astroturf. He might as well forget a rug.

But what if it made him feel better to have one on?

The hell with his feelings! What about mine? Putting a rug on me would be like first restoring my sight and then taking it away from me. I don't need that. I have my pride, you know. To tell you the absolute truth, I think Dick looks a hell of a lot better now than before. He'd look even better if he'd trim some of the stray hairs he's got up on top, and maybe give a little buff job to keep up the shine. But both of us look great this way. At least that's my opinion. You'd have to ask him what he thinks.

Just to play devil's advocate for a moment, Pate, what about when you sweat? There's no hair to catch it.

That's not a big deal. Dick's a couch potato. He doesn't sweat much.

Do you hope that Dick will one day shave his side and back hair off?

Do I? Of course. To frolic naked like the day I was born would be a real kick. Look, I've tried to reason with Dick. I once sent him a message that said, "Listen, you look like an ordinary bald guy this way. Every baldie has hair on the sides and in back. I'm not complaining, mind you, but the look is passé. Shave it all off. Do a Yul." Dick's a very indecisive guy. I know he likes the idea of being free from all hair worries. But he thinks a shaved head would make him stick out. I think it would distinguish him. Don't you think I want great-looking babes to come over and stroke me and tell Dick they've never seen anything so sensual and so cute? That's what happens. I'd have a personal look. I think it would be real bold. But Dick doesn't think so. Right now, it's a semantic argument. But I'll win out. I always do.

Thank you, Dick's Pate, it's been a pleasure.

No problem . . . Say, do I see the beginning of a bald spot in the back of your head?

What? Where?

Right here. Wait, let me give you a mirror.

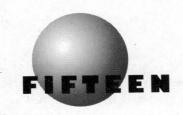

FIFTEEN

BALDNESS ON TELEVISION: THE MEDIUM SHOULD BE ASHAMED OF ITSELF

○

BALDMAN WATCHES a lot of television, but he's not always very happy about it. One morning, he turned on a rerun of *The Golden Girls* and this is what he got: oversexed Blanche Devereaux (Rue McClanahan) is in a terrible state. She has a recurring nightmare that she is caught in an enclosed space with a score of bald men. Doom will befall her. Then her worst dream comes true: She's on an airplane filled with unhaired guys like me. She panics, convinced that the true-life sight of a group of pilgarlics will send the plane crashing into the ocean. Her roommate Dorothy (Bea Arthur), whose ex-husband is bald and sports an obvious rug, tells her: "It's all right, Blanche. The captain just turned off the 'No Bald Men' sign." But Blanche's fears are unfounded: the fearsome troop of baldies she is convinced will crash the plane are actually en route to the Bahamas for a Mr. Clean reunion.

Is this any way to treat bald men? Does anybody on TV have bad dreams about men with pompadours? Did women awaken in a pool of sweat from nightmares about Ed "Kookie" Byrnes? Of course not. Such mistreatment of bald men is standard on television. How many times did the bewigged Carl Reiner, as Alan Brady in *The Dick Van Dyke Show*, run roughshod over Mel Cooley, his lackey brother-in-law/producer (played by the estimable Richard Deacon)? How many times did Alan tell Mel, "Shut up, Mel"? Remember when Buddy (Morey Amsterdam), the wisecracking comedy writer on Brady's show, said that Mel belonged to the FBI—Fat, Bald and Ignorant?

But is enough enough? Never on TV. The airwaves have hair. Check your antennas and cables for traces of split ends. Television is a vastly overhaired medium, aligned against us bald guys. The evidence is as plain as the nose on Jamie Farr's face. Not only are bald men conspicuously missing as series stars and network anchormen, but even when they are cast in major or supporting roles, they usually portray an odd lot of boobs, fools and second bananas. I've eliminated from consideration the bald stars who wear hairpieces, for these pseudo-haired believe (unfortunately, with good cause) that their survival on TV requires having a well-made rug. Captain Kirk, are you there?

There is the story of the TV studio chief and former network executive, who has an extraordinary hair obsession. He has two hairpieces. One is long and one is short. Some days he'll wear the long one and tell his secretary that he's going out for a haircut. Later that day, he'll return wearing the short one. It's no wonder that with pseudo-haired people like this guy bald men are abused on the tube.

There is overwhelming evidence of the prejudice against bald men. In the First Official Bald Man Survey of Baldness Bias on TV, I combed *The Complete Directory to Prime Time Network TV Shows*. Of the thousands of shows listed, I determined that 175 shows had casts that included bald men (not including guest starring roles by bald actors), but only 59 had bald stars or featured actors. And I regret to say that not all the stars were treated as they would if they had hair. Just witness the negative, unattractive images of bald men that TV has perpetrated.

None of this is meant to criticize the actors, who were only doing what was asked of them. It's not their fault they didn't get hired to play suave detectives, handsome romantic leads or TV anchormen. Rather, my criticism is of the producers, the hair-obsessed powers that be.

Actor	Role	Character Image
Jack Albertson	Ed Brown, *Chico and the Man*	Dyspeptic, carping, badly dressed garage owner who won't tell people he likes Chico; wore hat most of the time
Sorrell Booke	Boss Hogg, *The Dukes of Hazzard*	Moronic, semiliterate Southern sheriff
Edgar Buchanan	Uncle Joe, *Petticoat Junction*	Slothful hanger-on in rural hotel
Roger C. Carmel	Roger Buell, *The Mothers-in-Law* (replaced by Richard Deacon in second season; see: Richard Deacon)	Oddball, weak-willed TV writer
Richard Castellano	Joe Vitale, *Joe and Sons*, Joe Girelli *The Super*	Simple, fat factory worker Simple, fat superintendent
James Coco	Joe Dumpling, *The Dumplings*	Fat lunch counter owner with no upward mobility
Tim Conway	Rango, *Rango*	Inept, bumbling Texas Ranger
Jackie Coogan	Uncle Fester, *The Addams Family*	Ghoulish muu-muu wearer who lit light bulbs in his mouth

Actor	Role	Character Image
Richard Deacon	Mel Cooley, *The Dick Van Dyke Show*	Weak-willed sycophant glad to be abused by his coworkers and boss
Dom DeLuise	Stanley Belmont, *Lotsa Luck*	Menial bus-company worker who allows bum brother-in-law to sponge off him
Danny DeVito	Louie De Palma, *Taxi*	Cruel, overbearing miscreant taxicab dispatcher
Herb Edelman	Stanley Zbornack, *The Golden Girls*	Obnoxious, mooching ex-husband of Dorothy; wearer of bad wig
Dann Florek	Dave Meyer, *L.A. Law*	Obnoxious, boring, simpering direct-mail entrepreneur with amazingly low self-image
William Frawley	Fred Mertz, *I Love Lucy*	Tightwad landlord who insults and ignores his wife
Alan Funt	Host-creator, *Candid Camera*	Voyeuristic intruder into unsuspecting people's lives, often embarrassing them
Larry Gelman	Dr. Bernie Tupperman, *The Bob Newhart Show*	Nerdy, shleppy urologist

Actor	Role	Character Image
Sherman Hemsley	George Jefferson, *The Jeffersons*	Nouveau riche, egotistical, strutting, bigoted dry cleaner
Howard Hesseman	Dr. Johnny Fever, *WKRP in Cincinnati*	Brain-fried, freaked-out disc jockey
John Houseman	Charles Kingsfield, *The Paper Chase*	Imperious, harsh, elitist, heartless law professor
Gordon Jump	Arthur Carlson, *WKRP in Cincinnati*	Mama's boy ineptly running low-rated radio station
Werner Klemperer	Colonel Klink, *Hogan's Heroes*	Simpering Nazi POW camp commandant always outwitted by his prisoners
Don Knotts	Barney Fife, *The Andy Griffith Show*	Bumbling, inept, nervous, horny deputy sheriff
	Ralph Furley, *Three's Company*	Bumbling, inept, horny landlord with bad combover
Al Lewis	Grandpa Munster, *The Munsters*	Green, centuries-old vampire who could turn into a bat or a wolf
Gavin MacLeod	Merrill Stubing, *The Love Boat*	Cruise ship captain whose main job is to seat lonely old ladies at his table

Actor	Role	Character Image
Mr. Magoo	*The Famous Adventures of Mr. Magoo*	Absent-minded, myopic, eccentric millionaire; a menace on the road
Gerald McRaney	Rick Simon, *Simon & Simon*	Lazy, eccentric, grumpy half of fraternal detective team
Barry Morse	Lieutenant Gerard, *The Fugitive*	Humorless, no-nonsense detective who spends five years chasing an innocent man
Edward Platt	Thaddeus, the Chief, *Get Smart*	Leader of spy agency CONTROL who could not control, tame or fire boobish Maxwell Smart
Alan Rachins	Douglas Brackman, *L.A. Law*	Anal-retentive, skinflint law firm partner
Carl Reiner	Alan Brady, *The Dick Van Dyke Show*	Egotistical, insulting star with a deskful of toupees
Don Rickles	*C.P.O. Sharkey*	Shrill, insulting naval officer in perpetual bug-eyed state
Phil Silvers	Sergeant Ernie Bilko, *The Phil Silvers Show*	Scheming, loud con man in Midwestern Fort Baxter

Actor	Role	Character Image
David Ogden Stiers	Major Winchester, M*A*S*H	Pompous, selfish, overbearing surgeon who refused to fit into the M*A*S*H unit
Jeffrey Tambor	Alan Wachtel, *Hill Street Blues*	Transvestite criminal court judge
Vic Tayback	Diner-owner Mel on *Alice*	Greasy, foul exploiter of his waitresses
Abe Vigoda	Fish on *Barney Miller* and *Fish*	Dyspeptic, toilet-bound cop obsessed with his hemorrhoids
Ned Wertimer	Ralph the doorman, *The Jeffersons*	Nerdy sycophant willing to do any errand for a buck

This survey does not ignore some of the favorable images fostered by a smaller group of proud, bare-headed bald actors. Unfortunately, their ranks are much smaller.

Actor	Role	Character Image
Ed Asner	Lou Grant, *The Mary Tyler Moore Show, Lou Grant*	Soft-hearted grump with strong journalistic instincts in comedy and drama
Herschel Bernardi	Arnie Nuvo, *Arnie*	Earnest family man promoted to executive in a flange company

Actor	Role	Character Image
Yul Brynner	The King, *Anna and the King*	Imperious king of Siam
Michael Conrad	Sergeant Philip Esterhaus, *Hill Street Blues*	Caring, efficient administrator of station house given to torrid love affairs
William Conrad	Frank Cannon, *Cannon*	Overindulgent and obese but smart and dedicated private eye
Louis Gossett, Jr.	Fiddler, *Roots*	Sage, compassionate, intelligent slave
Norman Lloyd	Dr. Daniel Auschlander, *St. Elsewhere*	Wise and intelligent hospital physician dying of cancer
E. G. Marshall	Dr. David Craig, *The New Doctors*	Respected doctor dedicated to improving medical techniques
Gerald McRaney	Major MacGillis, *Major Dad*	Stouthearted Marine with a heart of gold who mellows when he marries liberal reporter
Richard Moll	Bull Shannon, *Night Court*	Kindly, shaved-headed court bailiff, often confused with a monster
Pernell Roberts	Dr. John McIntyre, *Trapper John, M.D.*	Suave superstar surgeon (redeeming himself from wearing rug on *Bonanza*)

Actor	Role	Character Image
Telly Savalas	Theo Kojak, *Kojak*	Strong, authoritative, lollypop-sucking detective, loath to use a gun
Willard Scott	Weatherman, *Today Show*	Kind, peaceful and charitable; spotlights good causes from places around the country

The history of television is filled with great leading men (James Arness, Robert Wagner, Jack Lord, Don Johnson, Alan Alda, Raymond Burr, James Garner, Michael Landon, Andy Griffith and Fred Flintstone), star comedians (Milton Berle, Jackie Gleason, Danny Thomas, Johnny Carson, Bill Cosby, Desi Arnaz and Richard Lewis), game show hosts (Tom Kennedy, Alex Trebek, Bill Cullen, Bob Barker, Geoff Edwards, Gene Rayburn and Peter Marshall) and anchormen (Edward R. Murrow, Walter Cronkite, Dan Rather, Chet Huntley, Peter Jennings, David Brinkley and Tom Brokaw).

History is less kind to the bald. Few bald men have been *the* stars of their shows, whether they projected positive or negative images. That is, unless you count the conga line of TV stars who have worn hairpieces to further their careers, men like Burt Reynolds, Stacy Keach, William Shatner, Ken Howard (who now goes without hair professionally), Jack Benny, George Burns, Howard Cosell, Dan Blocker (reportedly), Andy Williams, Lorne Greene and sportscaster Marv Albert (allegedly).

Of all the main "star" categories, bald anchormen are virtually an endangered species, although there were never many to start with. In my memory, the only balding star anchormen or newsmen have been Edwin Newman (who anchored a number of prime-time specials and filled in for regular anchors but succeeded most in his books and commentaries on language) and Charles Kuralt, who's never been the full-time anchor of a nightly newscast (only filling in for Dan Rather). Kuralt's two prime-time series (*On the Road* and *The American Parade*, which failed along with haired co-host Bill Moyers) fizzled and the gentle Southerner found permanent success only as the host of the CBS *Sunday Morning* program. Yes, early TV anchorman John Cameron Swayze (known best for his Timex "they take a licking but keep on ticking" commercials) was really bald, but he wore a hairpiece. Clearly, the TV powers don't mind age, wrinkles or gray hair, but put a *baldie* permanently behind the anchor desk and watch the light shine off his pate? Never!

As for bald game-show hosts—our jolly guides through trivia, cash, prizes and Dicker & Dicker of Beverly Hills—they are rare, too. Can you name one, besides Joe Garagiola (*To Tell the Truth* and *Sale of the Century*)? And this wasn't even Joe's real vocation, for he achieved true success elsewhere, as a sportscaster.

As I write this, I sense that there may be a ray of hope. Recently, there have been a number of bald stars populating TV, among them Telly Savalas (back for a season as *Kojak*), Bill Kirchenbauer (as the coach in *Just the Ten of Us*, a spinoff of the aggressively haired *Growing Pains*), Richard Moll (as Bull in *Night Court*), William Conrad (in *Jake and the Fat Man*), Patrick Stewart (in *Star Trek: The Next Generation*) and Joe Regalbuto, who, as Frank Fontana in *Murphy Brown*, plays a neat joke on antibaldness phobia in news by going bareheaded most of the time, but wearing a very obvious rug when he is an anchorman. It's also pleasant to see an urbane correspondent like the slowly balding Garrick Utley anchoring both the Sunday version of the *Today Show* and *Meet the Press*. But it is equally unpleasant to watch the sad progress of the TV career of the great shaved-headed actor Louis Gossett, Jr. Not one of his shows (*The Young Rebels, The Lazarus Syndrome, The Powers of Matthew Star* and *Gideon*) have ever lasted a year. *Gideon*, part of the rotating ABC

Saturday Night Movie, was replaced by the lustrously haired Jaclyn Smith show, *Christine Cromwell*. Need I say more?

All is not 100 percent rotten in the state of television baldness, however. There have been a handful of great moments of self-realization by bald characters, such as Bub's (William Frawley) in *My Three Sons* realizing that for all his attempts to grow hair (including the infamous "Scalper Dalper" and a toupee bought by grandson Chip and modeled from a swatch of the family dog's hair), nothing could change the reality of his bare head or the personality that went with that unhaired head. Even Chip realizes this, for as Bub prepares to wear the ridiculous rug on a date, Chip tells Bub, "Give her a chance to like you the way you are," adding later to the rest of his family that Bub didn't wear it because he "doesn't need it. He's doing okay without it." As does Baldman.

But Baldman's Greatest Moment in Bald TV occurred on September 15, 1965, in an episode of *The Dick Van Dyke Show*, titled, "Coast to Coast Big Mouth." Fans of the show will remember that the TV star whom Rob (Van Dyke) writes for, the ultraegotistical Alan Brady (Carl Reiner), is bald, but wears a toupee. Nobody on the outside knows this for certain, until Rob's wife, Laura (Mary Tyler Moore), is trapped into the admission on a TV game show. Later that day, Laura goes to Alan's office to apologize. She nervously enters. Alan is talking to the mannequin heads on his desk, each one topped with a different toupee. His injured ankle is propped on an open desk drawer. Here are some excerpts from the episode:

ALAN: Fellas, there she is. There's the little lady who put us out of business . . . Laura, what the heck are you doing here? If you like to see ruins, why don't you go to Greece?
LAURA: You're not ruined.
ALAN: You've got a big mouth. If you wanted a free rotisserie or a dryer, I'd have gotten it for you. I'd have gotten you a house, a showplace.

LAURA: I think you look very nice without your . . .

ALAN (angrily): Hair! Hair!

LAURA: I told Rob to tell you how nice and natural and warm you looked.

ALAN: Like a father figure.

LAURA: No, just the opposite.

ALAN: A bald mother figure . . . Why didn't you just tell me this in private?

LAURA: I didn't think it was the place.

ALAN: No, your place is on network television. (Alan piles one rug on top of another onto his head.) This is a cute one. I had this one made so people will say, "Alan, you're losing your hair." Or this one, I have for swimming. Or this one, so people say, "Alan, you need a haircut." What do you suggest I do with these?

LAURA: There must be some needy bald people.

ALAN: Needy bald people. (He pounds on one of his mannequin heads.) Laura, you're a nut.

(Rob enters, and the tide turns. You'll notice a change in Alan's attitude, toward true acceptance of his head.)

ROB: Why don't you tell me what you'd tell Laura.

ALAN: Rob, you're a beautiful girl. Let me finish, sweetheart. If I'd seen you one hour after the show, I'd kill you. But I've been thinking. It's interesting that you like me without my hair. Because my secretary does, too, and so does my wife. That's three in favor.

ROB: Well, I've always said I liked you bald.

ALAN: That's four. My butcher is five. The fact that five dumb-bells like me this way isn't the only reason I've decided to be adorable about this mess.

ROB: You're going to be adorable?

ALAN: This incident has taken a strain off my brain. It's tough keeping a secret like this, and now that it's out, I feel better.

LAURA: You mean, you're happy I told?

ALAN (seething): Happy . . . Yes, I'm happy!

LAURA: I'm happy, too.

ALAN: Are you happy?

ROB: Yes.

ALAN: Oh, happy days are here again! Look at it this way. I'm not twenty-nine anymore. I'm an established genius. If anything, my publicity man said my hair was holding me back. Sooner or later, it was bound to come out. This way, I'm getting a lot of sympathy, not to mention the publicity.

ROB: Honey, I'll bet you never thought it'd turn out this well.

LAURA: Never. Maybe I ought to go on television and tell them about your nose.

(Alan pounces out of his seat.)

ALAN: You told her about my nose?!?!?

LAURA: I've always said I liked you without your nose.

(Reprinted by permission of Calvada Productions. Copyright © 1965 by Calvada Productions.)

Sadly, there are too few moments such as this one. Even if the episode aired twenty-five years ago, it has reverberated inside the bare head of Baldman ever since. If a self-centered show-biz character like Alan Brady can attain self-realization and admit to the public that he is unhaired, then many more of us can. C'mon, Burt Reynolds, take off that graying rug! William Shatner, beam that wig away to another galaxy! Even Carl Reiner, who in real life seemed to switch between wearing and not wearing a toupee, depending upon his mood, seems to have opted for full-time baldness. His son, Rob, who was balding throughout much of *All in the Family* and covered up, is now a delightfully bald and bearded film director of great repute (*When Harry Met Sally* and others) who thinks hair replacements are "so bad, so dumb, much dumber than the guy without hair."

The lesson of Alan Brady and Bub is that we are not ourselves when we don psuedo-hair, which tells the story of Baldman's life pretty succinctly. With false hair, we project a false image. We are worshiping false idols when we wear wigs. Few friendlier probald words were uttered by a haired TV character than those from Fred MacMurray, as Steve Douglas in *My Three Sons*, when he explained hair's role in our society to his son Chip: "Most people accept a man for what he is, hair or no hair."

The bald gods now rest a little more comfortably.

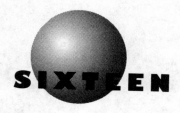

SIXTEEN

JOHN CAPPS AND THE CULT OF THE BALD

THE THIRTY-NINE-SEAT PLANE has just landed in New Bern, North Carolina. My buddy Steve and I expect to be met by somebody from the Bald-Headed Men of America to take us to their sixteenth annual convention.

"I hope whoever's there isn't walking around with a sandwich sign that says, 'Howdy baldies!' " Steve says.

"I just hope they recognize us," I say.

"How could they miss? We're the only two bald guys on the plane," says Steve.

Waiting to meet us, with two small signs, is Lee Capps, brother of Bald-Headed Men of America founder John Capps.

Lee is wearing a BHMA cap, which I assume covers a bare pate.

"What are you hiding there?" I ask.

"My hair," he says, lifting the cap sheepishly. Lee's a black sheep in the presence of brother John, who insists that Lee's hair is thinner than he lets on.

"There are five generations of baldness in our family," Lee says, "and when I was in high school, my hair started falling out in clumps. I just thought I'd be bald, but it grew back."

While Lee waited for us, he says, a woman in her twenties spotted him wearing a T-shirt that said: "Rub a Bald Head Tonight."

"I just have to have that," she said. "I'll give you twenty dollars."

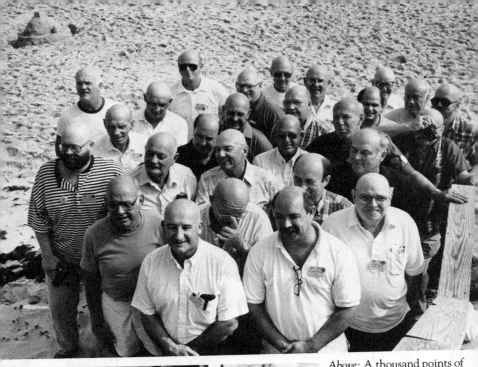

Above: A thousand points of light illuminate the convention's official board meeting.

Photo by Baldman

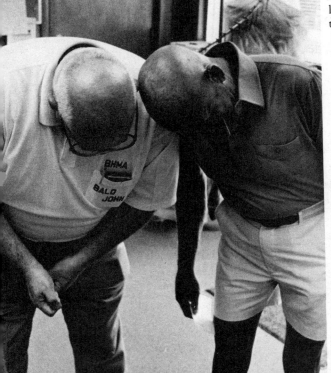

Left: John Capps (left), head head of the Bald-Headed Men of America, and John Wood (right) demonstrate the no-hair-in-the-eyes putting stroke, which doubles as the correct method of prayer to the Great God Yul Brynner.

Photo by Baldman

"But I won't have a shirt," said Lee.

"I'll give you my husband's," she countered.

Lee made the deal—a good one, since the shirts costs five dollars at the convention—and greets us in a striped shirt with the name "Bill" stitched above the pocket.

Lee wanted to bring his bald father-in-law along, but his mother-in-law balked.

"He's got the perfect head for baldness," says Lee. "She says he doesn't need to use up his vacation time with a bunch of bald men."

We drive the half-hour to the convention in the official Bald-Headed Men of America van.

"I've spent fifteen years waiting for my hair to fall out," he says. "I'm still waiting."

My wait ended years ago.

Mickey Mantle was my first hero, followed by Willis Reed, Joe Namath and Gay Talese. As I got older and balder, my worship gravitated toward Yul Brynner. My new hero is John T. Capps III, a beefy, working-class guy with a thick Carolina drawl and a resemblance to Uncle Fester of *The Addams Family* (without, of course, the black muu-muu and the light bulb in his mouth). As head head of the BHMA, John runs the only organization I belong to, a group of which I can truly proclaim: "These are my people."

John Capps is the Lenin of us bald Bolsheviks, a hairless revolutionary in the vanguard of the Bald Generation. He prays, he gives time to civic causes and he's a Rotarian. His secretary, Barbara Walton, brags that he's the kind of guy who once gave stuck-in-traffic drivers things to do while they waited for the drawbridge between Morehead City and Atlantic Beach to open. Capps moves with surprising ease, as if his head gives him greater aerodynamism. He bounds around like a man with deep faith in his mission, a Jimmy Carter for the hairless.

John sports a nubby fringe of gray stubble around his chubby dome and a yellow pullover shirt with "Bald John" stitched in black letters on his pocket. He founded the Bald-Headed Men of America in Dunn, North Carolina, and for a while considered holding his annual conventions on Baldhead Island, but the snotty developers thought a bunch of baldies was too low-rent for their hoity-toity time-share vacationers. He eventually moved to Morehead City, a serendipitous relocation that supplies an endless number of bad jokes and the perfect newspaper dateline. John calls his bald Eden "More Head (Less Hair) City." Some people in town support what he does, others think he's a bit deranged. But nearly all four thousand year-round residents, he says, know who Bald John is.

Capps's first words to me come in a pleasant bellow-drawl: "C'mon, bring your bald head over here."

"C'mon, bring your bald head over here."

Anyplace else, that would bring the speaker my knee in his gut. I'm not partial to being called "baldie" by someone with hair, but this is, after all, the Dome Capital, where "Hey baldie" is a term of endearment that spurs *everybody* to turn as one with a smile on his face. If you don't like being tagged a chrome dome at the Bald-Headed Men's yearly confab, you might as well enlist in Sy Sperling's Army of Hair Weaves.

John issues his invitation as I enter the Holiday Inn in Atlantic Beach, a bridge-span away from Morehead City. I don't know what comes first: his words or seeing all those bald heads in the lobby posing for a Philadelphia TV station. An octet of early arriving conventioneers are posing before a wall-length mirror, bald heads thrust forward, hands smoothing over domes in unison. It's very raucous and very silly, like standing beside Ralph Kramden and Ed Norton as they cast their fishing poles off Fred's Landing, but a shade more significant.

If I am ever to fulfill my role as Baldman, I reckon, I have to be silly. I have to join this hairless hootenanny.

"Lots of glare coming off us," I say to John Kiefer, as we both looked at our reflections in the mirror.

"Hey, watch that!" he says, half-serious.

"That's something only one baldie can say to the other," I say.

"Sure," says Kiefer, "you're right."

"We're all brothers here," I tell him.

The camera rolls, and John exhorts us to chant the traditional Bald-Headed Men benediction:

"Hip, hip. Bald is beautiful. Bald is beautiful. Bald is beautiful."

Capps goes to the phone to talk to a reporter. Reporters love Capps. After sixteen years of conventions, they keep calling him for bits of cornpone Baldosophy. Capps will stop the convention for any reporter, photographer or film crew, figuring that if he cooperates, he'll charm anyone into good public relations.

"This is the Head Head from Morehead," he tells the reporter on the phone. "We're head-to-head in Morehead, lookin' for the perfect head."

Standing apart from the ceremony's opening ceremonies is my friend Steve. He balded before I did, and now we're equally hairless, a fact he is loath to admit. His excuse is that his bald spot is too small to make him a baldie, a claim that has been demonstrably false for ten years. Capps has seen people like Steve, members of the Silent Baldority who suffer in silence.

"C'mon over, Steve," roars Capps.

"No, no, I'll just stay right here," says Steve, standing implacably by the registration desk. He fears that if any of his business customers in North Carolina see him in any photos or TV footage, his credibility may suffer. But how serious could the damage be from his customers, who buy Steve's laundry bags and toilet seats?

On the other hand, Steve is one of the silliest people I know. After knowing him for twenty years, I'm certain that his loyalties are torn. And Capps's confidence in converting him to one of his own is unflappable.

"By Sunday," Capps predicts, "he'll be as bald as the rest of us."

Extraordinary roles sometimes present themselves to ordinary men. That's how bald activism came to John Capps. Baldness came to John early in life, just as it had to his daddy and his daddy's daddy. Being bald was as natural as breathing in the Capps family.

"My hair started departing when I was fifteen," says John. "As a fourth generation of baldness, I had a positive attitude at home. I never encountered a problem. I made up the nickname 'Bald John.' Being involved in high school political campaigns, with two or three Johns running, it was easy to say, 'Vote for Bald John, He Won't Put Anything Over Your Eyes.' I'd run up and down the basketball court and people would cheer for 'Bald John.'

"It set me apart, gave me individuality. I never got turned down for a date because I was baldheaded. At least not as far as I knew. If a girl was May Day Queen, I'd call her up for a date. If she was homecoming queen and I wasn't dating her, I'd call her up for a date."

Hairlessness in 1950s and 1960s North Carolina made no difference, even to the youthful John Capps. He graduated high school and worked his way through eight years of college with a tobacco company that promoted him in part because of the maturity imparted by his bare head.

It wasn't until 1973, when he sought a sales job with a financial printer, that haired prejudice reared its ugly head.

"They turned me down for the job because I didn't have hair on my head," says John. "That's what they told me. They said they specifically wanted a young, fresh, dynamic approach. It stunned me to know that the way I looked had more impact than what I was. It's like they had an image that hair was part of the dress-for-success uniform. I didn't say much. I just thanked them for their time and left. Remember, this was before anybody really thought about suing for discrimination like this. I thought it was company policy. Why question it?

"But then I made a decision," he continues. "I was young and dynamic and wanted to be in a leadership role. So I started the Bald-Headed Men of America in Dunn. We had four people at the first convention, including my uncle Bob."

The BHMA is low-keyed. It doesn't advertise or rent out its mailing lists. It doesn't chase for members. If someone wants information, Capps sends it. But there's not much follow-up. I sense that Capps doesn't want the organization to get too big or bureaucratic or out of his control lest it lose its genteel charm.

Whatever he has done works. The conventions are fun, the media coverage startlingly positive. Capps has taken his bald shtick on the road to Johnny Carson, Ted Koppel and Phil Donahue. Erma Bombeck wrote about him and Charles Kuralt profiled him.

"The media love us because they know we'll cooperate with them," says Capps. "Where else are they going to get fifty bald guys to do whatever they ask, and sometimes more?"

Bald evangelism has paid off in twenty thousand members for the BHMA (though only a small fraction are paying members) and regular attendance of about fifty baldies and their families at each convention.

"John," I say, "fifty doesn't sound like too many people."

"People are hung up on numbers, and we don't even count how many we get," he tells me. "We just say we've got a nice roomful of heads. Have you ever been to a hairy convention? If hair is so popular or in vogue, why isn't there a big hair convention for all the hairy people in America?"

Why indeed?

The rare criticism Capps gets for his efforts is from people who allege that he singles baldies out for ridicule rather than encouraging us to seek alternatives to hairlessness. Don't echo those negatives to Capps's loyal legion of heads. We don't feel stigmatized or ridiculed even if we don't all agree with John that being bald is the greatest thing in the world. We agree when he says, "We have no room for plugs, rugs or drugs."

My admiration for him took a quantum leap when he told me that in 1988, the company that makes a hair growth potion, the Helsinki Formula, tried to horn in on the convention. They wanted to put up a counter-display of the formula in the Holiday Inn lobby to compete with Capps's probald shirts, combs, bumper stickers, videos, coffee mugs and pennants. Capps said no. So the company said it wanted to picket outside the hotel, but neither the hotel nor the counties who control different parts of the land on which the hotel stands would stand for it.

Undaunted, the company rented an airplane to drag a banner saying: "Real Men Don't Go Topless. Use the Formula." It was a bit of a hoot for the townsfolk, and the local papers played it up: a little bit of controversy put some hair on the issue.

"I was upset," Capps says, "that the good works and positive mental attitude that this association has would be questioned or jeopardized by someone who's never been a part of it, but only wanted to use it for individual, selfish gain. They just said, 'Hey, this is a heck of an idea to get promotion for our business.' I don't think it was the Christian thing to do."

Capps has plenty of followers. He's a natural leader: inspiring, humorous, well-organized, humble and religious (saying grace precedes each convention meal and its awards fete). He has spawned true-believing zealots of the cause—baldies who long ago accepted their unhaired utopia. They're not Rambos, but then, have you seen Sylvester Stallone's hair? Way too much. The Bald-Headed Men deplore excess, in any form.

If Capps had to assemble an army to slay the haired, Walter Jackson would lead the charge. Walter's fully shaven head is a work of tonsorial art. It is the perfect head for baldness: round, unblemished, without bumps or scars. His only facial hair resides above his upper lip. He has been bald since he was a teenager; he looked so much older than his years that his future mother-in-law couldn't believe he was twenty-one and tried to stop him from dating his wife-to-be, Vicki. At age fifty, the ex-trucker and ex-Marine owns a commercial cleaning business that he calls "Mr. Clean and His Machine." He answers to the name Mr. Kojak. Listen to Walter, and you ascend quickly into the Bald New World.

"Being bald is one of the cleanest feelings in the world," says Walter. "When I don't shave my head for a few days, I can't wait to get to that razor. Ahhhhh! It's like when you're a kid playin' nekkid in the fields and the wind hits your buttocks."

"Being bald has been a real gain for me. I don't think people would accept me being hairy. I introduce myself as 'Kojak, King of the Bald.' I think when people see something real clean, they trust it. Cleanliness is next to Godliness. People put you next to the Bible and God when you're bald. I think there's a special glow about people like us. I really believe if I had hair, people wouldn't trust me as much as they do. It's my drawing card."

Harold Fleischman is another kind of Capps foot soldier. Not possessed of Jackson's flair or independence, Harold is an example of the emotional handiwork of the Bald-Headed Men of America. Harold is sixty-nine years old, and in 1951, his hair fell out within three weeks of getting an allergy shot. Not only was he deprived of the hair on his head, but nary a hair, a fingernail or toenail was left on his entire body. It was as if he returned to the womb, and he awaited maturity where his hair would regenerate. But it did not. Not a hair has grown ever since, and one could say that Harold never accepted his loss until he discovered Capps.

"I was thirty-one and it was traumatic," says Harold, who

lives in Greeneville, Tennessee. "I was an usher in a church, and I felt every eye was on me. The tears rolled out of my eyes. But I couldn't shoot myself."

Wife Dorothy adds, "He had beautiful blondish-red hair, and a red wavy beard. I felt real badly for him when he lost it. I was embarrassed. My mother-in-law was embarrassed. And I resented people staring. When I saw 'em looking, I'd look back until they moved their eyes."

Harold was passing through the BHMA's birthplace in Dunn, North Carolina, in 1978 when he saw a notice about the group, but he paid little heed to it. Over the years, he thought about it, but it wasn't until 1986 that he read an article about it in a senior citizens' magazine. In 1987, he attended the convention, and to no one's surprise, won the Smoothest Head Award. He now declines entry into the competition, graciously opening the door for other clean, buffed pates.

Thus began Harold's rebirth: interviews with him appeared in his hometown newspaper and forty other domestic and foreign newspapers, *Stars and Stripes* and *The Star*. He popped up on Phil Donahue's show and almost got on Dolly Parton's variety show. When Harold comes to the convention, he totes homemade easels to display his clippings. In the trunk of his car he always carries stacks of BHMA newsletters and sign-up sheets. He is a one-man, smooth-headed, horn-rimmed BHMA recruitment office.

Harold loves to relate the story of his post-BHMA life so much that he spends much of the weekend buttonholing anyone who will listen. "I say to Harold," Dorothy says, "tell people three stories. Any more, they get bored. Sometimes he listens, sometimes he doesn't."

Harold likes to say that ever since John Capps came into his life, "I've lived a life of notoriety."

Harold is no John Gotti in the notoriety department, but he shines in his own particular way. "When you realize that

Harold was about physically and mentally destroyed, this put a whole new purpose in his life," says Capps. "You see him today and you have more respect for him. What other organization can you see that does this? Even if he tells the same stories all the time, like my daddy."

There aren't many gatherings where the appearance of the people automatically connotes their unity. Unless Elks or Shriners or Raccoons wear their hats, you don't know if they're part of a group or not. But let loose fifty baldies at once on a hotel with a few haired folk, and you sense that this might be a reunion of Mr. Cleans.

A young burr-headed Marine is on the lobby phone. He knows what's going on, but doesn't fully comprehend it.

"You won't believe it," he says. "This place is filled with bald guys. They're everywhere. I mean it. Everybody is bald."

This convention would do Norman Vincent Peale and Dale Carnegie proud. My people are devout converts to the bald cause. They believe that bald is best, and who am I to argue? Only a couple seem anywhere near ambivalent, but by weekend's end, they will be complete devotees.

Capps is characteristically positive. "If we help just one person who came here sittin' on the fence, we're happy," he says, "and I know one who was helped the minute he sat down with us."

The happy testimonials come fast and furious, no matter where I go. In the hotel lobby, at Capps's house, at restaurants, by the pool—I get a sense of joyous group therapy, as if every bald guy came off his analyst's couch completely cured of the prohair neurosis. Everybody's got their war stories, but all say they've either always accepted their loss or gradually came to like it.

Ex-Marine John Wood long had a close crewcut. In the Second World War and the Korean War, he and his men shaved their heads "for luck." When he retired, his hair was almost gone, so he shaved off what was left. He's proud of winning the BHMA's '87 Solar Dome Award for the best-tanned dome. He says he spent the months before the convention working on his head's tan so he could win another Solar Dome, but in the last days, his skin peeled. "Most of us guys accept it," he says. "We think it's great."

Bob Procter, Capps's seventy-four-year-old uncle, has been bald for fifty years. He remembers his hair as well as Capps's blond tresses. "Back then," he says, "it never occurred to anybody that being bald was a problem. I just sweep it back and let it flow."

Walt Reidi, an ex–Sears Roebuck executive, says: "About seventeen years ago, I was bald on top. My wife was clipping my hair and I told her to cut it down more and more. So she went

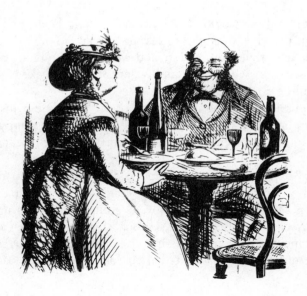

all the way, shaved it all off. Clean is mean. Hair is dirty. It never bothered me and it never bothered my wife."

Walt adds that he does have one problem with his Mr. Clean coiffure. "Perspiration," he says. "There's nothing to catch it. So I wear sweatbands underneath."

"Your head," cooes Walt's wife, Lupa, "gets kissed all the time."

John Ward has been bald for more than forty years and claims never to look in a mirror. "My father had hair when he died and he was eighty. My daddy's brothers all razz me, that I'm the baldest Ward they've ever seen. It's so easy [to care for] that I carry my razor in the car and shave there. I've worn out a dozen Norelcos."

Irv Brockington, a thirty-three-year-old insurance adjustor from Philadelphia, was a high school prankster and for several years felt someone was playing a twenty-four-hour-a-day practical joke on him by making him bald. But when he discovered that it wasn't a problem, he took steps to debunk the negative myths about baldness. Irv was soon on his way to being a fully evolved bald man.

"When I couldn't accept it," Irv says, "I must have had hundreds of hats. I even had hats with a duckbill. Then I threw most of them away. I went cold turkey, I went to the Betty Ford Bald Clinic. I realized it wasn't a real problem. When I started working for CIGNA, at my first meeting with my supervisor, I said, 'I'll never get mad enough to lose my hair over anything.' "

Mark Adams was born to be bald. If he had been a ten-year-old baldie, he would have enjoyed it. He was a teenage pilgarlic and at age twenty-five, he told his barber: "Cut it off! Cut it all off!"

"I love it," he says. "I'm a salesman. And I found out people remembered me because I'm bald. It's better than knowing me as the guy with warts. It never bothered me. My parents died when I was young and my grandparents raised me. Grandpa was bald. So were my uncles. . . . When I introduce myself at sales calls, I say, 'I'm your Bald Sometal Parts Salesman.' It really breaks the ice and people sure remember it. It's the power of positive thinking. I see guys who look like me and it bothers them. It's all in their head. Look, if we're all created in God's image, then God or his ancestors must have been bald. I always say I'm a solar collector for a sex machine."

One of the reporters at the convention is Mike Buchanan, a part-time anchorman with WUSA-TV in Washington, D.C. Mike shows up in a tattered brown pullover with a T-shirt showing underneath. He's got some hair up front, but a generous bald spot shines in back. Buchanan shed his objectivity completely, for he knows that reveling is more appropriate to the story than cogent analysis.

Buchanan stands amid us in a group shot at one point on Saturday and exhorts us.

"You guys ever hear of Rogaine?"

"No!" we shout.

"You guys ever hear of toupees?"

"No!"

"You guys ever hear of transplants?"

"No!"

Somebody shouts to him: "You ever hear of Gillette?"

"No!" screams Buchanan.

He assures us this will all go over well, if a bit strangely, on the following Monday's newscast.

A lot of bald guys are walking around the hotel with lipstick on their shiny heads on convention Saturday. The deep-red smacks upon the domes are the signs that they've been through the judging for the BHMA's Most Kissable Bald Head Award. Seven judges spend an hour rating the bussability of forty naked pates. But the judges are not just after the Kissability Quotient: awards will also be bestowed upon the smoothest, brownest, prettiest, most distinguished, tallest, shiniest and best all-around bald heads. There are also awards for bald lookalikes.

The contests were the only scheduled events of each convention until 1986 when sessions featuring the men talking about accepting their baldness and the women describing Life With Baldie were added. The gabfests, though not solemn, gave substance to what would seem the silliest gathering this side of Shriners and their water balloons. But the contests serve a Baldosophy tenet: that we must shed the negative vanity that comes from being bald, a vanity imposed on us by a hair-crazed society. Haired folk may think us daft, but then, we think they're overdressed.

So there are seven Southern women kissing and rubbing one bald head after another in a crowded hotel room.

"Ummm, I can't wait to kiss your bald heads!" exclaims the perpetually sunny Carol Tunstall, a striking nurse and model.

"We can be bribed," says Vicki Jackson.

I don't think this is what the Beach Boys had in mind when they immortalized Southern girls and the way they kissed, which kept their boyfriends warm at night. There's not much romance in this kind of kissing, There is a lot of blushing, though. Usually, the women approach the man from behind, hold his head in place and plant a big red one on his pate. Then they rub, observe and ask questions.

"Has anyone ever called you bad names?" Carol congenially asks me.

"The usual. Chrome dome and baldie," I reply.

"How did it make you feel?"

"Awful."

"Has anyone told you you looked like someone famous?" she asks.

"No."

"Well, thank you for letting me kiss your head," she says before moving to the next head.

Navy chief petty officer James Gafner is getting the treatment from Donna Bowdish, whose husband manages the hotel we're in. Donna strokes Gafner's fully shaved dome and likes it. A lot. Not everybody thinks a shiny top like Gafner's is worth admiring. According to Gafner's haired son, Travis, there was the time Gafner was on his ship and a helicopter attempting to land radioed down to "tell that bald guy to put someone on his head, it's causing us too much glare."

"Girls," says Donna, "can we have a smoothness test?"

Six judges at once planted their heads on Gafner's head, and seemed to be in some kind of scalpular orgasmic ecstasy.

I sneak a peak at their judging sheets and hear them talk. As Jim walks away, I tell him, "You're a lock for best all-around. They loved you." He smiles sheepishly.

I ask Donna to analyze the smoothness of la tete de Gafner.

"I was really impressed. There was a slight stubble to the right and left," she said.

"Doesn't that cut down on the smoothness?" I ask.

"No, you have to rub all over," she says. "And he's smooth. But remember, some stubble is unbelievably smooth, too.

"Each head," she says, "is its own individual thrill."

Eileen Gafner, James's wife, confides in me that she "likes showing James off. It's like having a mirror with me all the time. When I met him, he had a little hair, but then it started falling out rapidly. Then he came back from a cruise without any hair at all. It was a bit of a shock. The cat didn't like it at all. And the neighborhood kids started calling him Mr. Raisin Head."

The awards ceremony has all the bonhomie of a Rotary meeting, but add a prayer for Grace to the pot. Capps is the chief Rotarian, dispensing jokes, homilies and group announcements.

The lucky winners and runners-up stand on stage, waiting for Capps's instructions.

"Turn to your right," he says to one group, as they pose for photographers. "Turn to your left. Show us your best side."

The Smoothest Bald Head competition requires a four-headed "rub-off."

"You can tell the seasoned judges," says Capps, "by the way they go straight for the cranium."

One head, Jim Ross, a hospital worker in Louisville, Kentucky, who came here to the absolute disbelief of his colleagues, asks the judges, "Was it as good for you as it was for me?"

The winner, Newton Cummings, the first-ever Indian to attend a convention, weeps at the podium. He can only say, "I hope I can come back again."

The Most Kissable award requires a kiss-off, eventually won by easy-to-blush Steve Comer, whose red face approaches the color of his beard. He once had waist-length hair.

"My bald spot was never that noticeable until three or four years ago," he says. "I saw some photographs where the back of my head looked like a yarmulke. The receding hairline and my bald spot had met. So I shaved it all off. When I made that decision, I sent in my application to the Bald-Headed Men of America."

Comer advises Mr. Clean Wannabes: "I use barber's clippers and an electric razor to shave my head. The critical thing is to apply baby oil afterward to avoid diaper rash."

I am at the hotel bar with my friend, Steve, and another baldie, Paul T. (not his real name), who came equipped with a battery of camera equipment. Everywhere we went, Paul was sure to go. I mention that for this book, I'll need photographs of bald men.

"I have a collection of bald men photos," he says enthusiastically. "I have some of it here."

Paul returns with ten albums of five-by-seven photographs, filled with the images of anonymous bald guys.

"You're the first people to see these," he says.

"Oh."

Steve and I leaf through the pages.

"Is that Marvin Hagler?" I ask.

"No."

"Is that Hurricane Carter?" I ask.

"No."

"Is that Bud Collins?" I ask.

"No."

Paul stalks Philadelphia, snapping shots of bald men, mostly without their knowledge. Sometimes he'll meet a man on his rounds as a messenger and ask to take his picture for what he says is his private collection. Mostly, though, he is armed with a long zoom lens, waiting for baldies to stop at traffic lights. There are baldies separated by types and race: white, white with beard, fully shaved white; black, black with beard, fully shaved black.

"This . . . is a little strange," I say.

"It's different," he admits. "I've kept it private. None of my family knows about this."

Capps joins us.

"John," I say. "Paul has a collection of pictures of bald guys."

John looks through them. In disbelief, he says, "That's your hobby? Taking pictures of baldies?"

"Yes," Paul says shyly.

"That's weird," says Capps. "That's really weird."

Capps looks tired, feeling the strain of his Bald Marathon. Being the bald equivalent of Mao Zedong is tough business—all that dispensing of hairless wisdom can fatigue a man. So he's plunked down on a couch in the BHMA's hospitality suite. His mouth is in overdrive even if his usual bounce is in reserve.

"Bald guys who don't accept it have to get their minds straight," he says. "They have to believe in themselves. The cliché is it's mind over matter; it doesn't matter if the person doesn't really mind. Steve's a good example. He's gotten over the fact that he's not bald. On Friday he wasn't bald. His involvement in

Forest Hills, New York, told him it's a stigma to be baldheaded so he has a few extra cultivated strands on his head."

If there were a miracle cure, John is asked, that could give you hair without pain or risk, would you do it?

"I think that would make baldness more acceptable," he says, "because then folks like me who enjoy being bald would have an easy option. I wouldn't use it. I don't think everybody wants to look like everybody else. Your media market tells you how to look and dress. Group theory won over individuality and everybody thinks they have to have hair.

"Maybe we need a new direction and a bald head to lead the way. Look at our great bald leaders: George Washington, Booker T. Washington, Cyrus Vance McCormick. Who needs hair?"

At the tiny New Bern airport, we are waiting to board the plane when Capps, who had brought us there and left, returns with his instamatic camera.

"One more shot," he says. "Show me your heads!"

As he walks away, we chant, "Hip, hip. Bald is beautiful, bald is beautiful . . ."

The Wit and Wisdom
of
John Capps

Baldness is just mind over matter. It doesn't really matter if the person doesn't mind.

We don't have time for rugs, plugs or drugs.

If you don't got it, flaunt it.

The Lord is just, the Lord is fair. He gave some brains, the others hair.

Skin is in.

The great thing about being bald is when you putt, your hair doesn't fall in your eyes.

What brings us together is what we don't have. We bask in the sunshine. We don't miss a thing—even our hair.

It's a major change in a person's life, when after buying shampoo all that time, he has to buy Drano.

About all you can put your hair in is a cigar box. The only thing to stop hair from falling is the floor.

If you go five inches back from your eyebrows and you have no hair there, then your hair is waving goodbye.

Hang out with bald guys, you won't get in your wife's hair.

A Little Ode

On the head of us men who are bald,
   There is heaped a lot of abuse
But as our age advances, our hair
   Turns gray, or else it turns loose.

We stumble along on our wayward course,
   Through this world of toil and sin;
And our forehead grows long, our eyes
   Grow dim and our hair gets tattered and thin.

We've heard that it's 'cause "the grass
   Can't grow on a busy street";
There's the snide remark that the
   Cause is due to "thickness of the head's concrete."

These cutting remarks are enough
   To cause a siege of apoplexy,
But then we read that a shiny dome
   Is a sure sign a bald man is sexy.

It's a mark of distinction if upon our
   Head, we haven't any hair.
It sets us apart from all those fuzzy folks;
   It makes you suave and debonair.

The prettiest things we'll ever see,
   Are not always lean and mean.
There's a lot to be said for Yul Brynner . . .
   An onion . . . and Mr. Clean.

So we'll comb our hair with a washrag,
   And no worry about the glare,
If a fly slides down and breaks his leg,
   Yet we'll not despair.

Though the mockers call us "Slick" or "Curly,"
  We'll take it with a grin,
'Cause we've got a crown of distinction . . .
  A headpiece . . . made out of skin!

                              —adapted by John Capps
                              (author unknown)

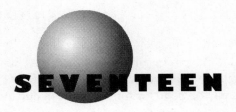

SEVENTEEN

NOW, AS A PUBLIC SERVICE, BALDMAN BUYS A HAIRPIECE

○

Maury Povich: Baldman—unhaired activist—or false-haired fraud? We follow him as he buys a hairpiece at this posh midtown toupee parlor . . . A Current Affair has exclusive footage of Baldman, footage that he has sued to stop us from showing. Sorry, Baldman, here's our hair-raising story—Your Cheatin' Scalp. [Ka-chungggg!]

ON A GRAY November day, I confess, I went to buy a hairpiece. Now, wait a minute! Don't go pulling my fringe hair out! Buying a rug is a public service, not an act of betrayal. I've witnessed hair transplants, visited the evil empire of minoxidil and yakked with Sy Sperling. For me to know about hairpieces, I felt I had to get one to see what the world thinks.

Think of me as the bald George Plimpton, going out in the world of hair replacement much as Plimpton did in trying out as a Detroit Lions quarterback and a Boston Bruins goalie to find out what their worlds were like. He didn't stay in those worlds; he merely visited them.

I had to know what it was like to be a rugster—and doing this was far easier than smearing minoxidil on my head for a year, getting a weave or going under the knife for a transplant. I was fated to buy a hairpiece so I could accurately report to my constituency about these issues: How does it feel? What do people who know me think about it? Are people who don't know me laughing and pirouetting to see how bad it is? Will it change me? Will I be paranoid?

I'm paying $850 for this test, so I'm putting my money where my scalp is.

Guys—This Rug's For You.

THE MEASUREMENT

Which hairmeister should I bring my head to? Those I encountered during my undercover work (see "Dear Yul: Diary of a Bald Man") were a mixed bag of the absurd, the smooth, the insulting and the patronizing. But who was my friendliest, most cost-effective enemy? Whom could I trust to produce a wall-to-wall scalp rug that wouldn't look like Howard Cosell's oversized piece and would provide me with a human laboratory for attitudes toward the false-haired me?

I choose Louis of Hairlines International. Why? He was not expensive. He didn't trash his competitors even when I prodded him. He spent the most time with me during a free consultation. Plus, he seemed stylish. I want someone with talent; I don't want to walk around with the kind of piece I saw on my summer camp arts-and-crafts counselor, whom we nicknamed "Toupee Away."

The measurement process is a high-tech wonder. Louis lays a strip of Saran Wrap (freezer strength, I hope) around the circumference of my pate. I feel like a bowl of leftover asparagus. He stretches the wrapping tautly over my tundra.

Louis secures the wrapping with Scotch tape, as the low-tech mold of my scalp starts to take form. Every inch of the wrap is now covered with strips of tape.

"Is this special hairpiece tape?" I ask.

"Just the regular kind," Louis says, with a faint chuckle.

With a green marker, Louis starts drawing around the circumference of the mold. I'm glad Louis is doodling on the tape and Saran Wrap, not on my tender scalp.

At about this time, I flip out my Vivitar instamatic camera. I ask if Louis or his assistant, Guy, could snap some shots so I would have a record of the process. After a long pause (he knows I am a writer; does he suspect me of being undercover Baldman?), Louis grumbles his assent and Guy comes in. Guy is excited. He thinks all victims should have their pictures taken so there'd be a chronicle of all the *faux* hair foisted on their clients. Guy, a curly-haired (perhaps berugged) guy with a big black mustache, delightedly snaps a few shots.

Louis then snips two locks from the back of my head and tapes them to the mold.

Then he removes the mold and places a black hairpiece on my head, a model for the piece he will design for me. It gives me nearly a full head of false hair with slight recessions on the sides of my frontal hairline. He combs it down, spritzes it a bit and blends the piece with my own hair.

I have the same reaction as I did with all the hairpieces I tried on during my research: however much hair now sits upon my pate, I still see the pate in my bald's-eye. I see skin where other men see hair.

Louis proceeds. He refines the mold by cutting it to the measurements provided by the model piece he had plopped on my head.

"Mine will look like that?" I ask.

"Sure, but the color will be lighter to match yours."

"Will it be real hair?"

"If you want it," says Louis. "But real hair oxidizes faster."

"I want real."

I don't do AstroTurf.

Step one is now over. Now I have a six-week wait until the stork delivers my piece.

THE GUILT

I'm looking at a picture of myself with the test toupee Louis tried on me. This is the stiffest test yet presented to Baldman. I won't say that I look good with it. Not that I don't think I look good bald, but the piece gives my head an even, symmetrical look and a pretty good profile. Of course, if I shave my beard and fringe hair off, I'd have a symmetrical look, too. But then, so did eggheaded Orson Welles when he played the aged Citizen Kane.

But here's my dilemma: What do I do if I get the piece and I like it so much that I really *want* to wear it all the time? Surely, this would be an act of scalpist treason. This book would be a complete lie and I would be made out to be a fake-haired fool. The Page Six gnomes of the *New York Post* would stalk me, waiting for the moment when Baldman showed his true follicles and went about his regular life with a wig that only a mother (of the woman whose hair I'd be wearing) could love.

I find myself wondering if there is a statute of limitations on being Baldman. Do I have to wait one, two or three years after the publication of this book before I can wear the rug full-time? If I ignore the statute of limitations, will I have to surrender all royalties to a bald tribunal?

No, no, no. I must be firm. No matter how much I may like my bewigged look, I shall defend the honor of Baldman and bald men around the world. Once I finish my field work, I shall stow my wig away in a dark, warm drawer, letting it die a slow death on a mannequin head. Or maybe I'll give it away to some needy bald person.

BALDMAN'S SCALP HELD HOSTAGE

Louis calls. The hairpiece has landed. I repeat my mantra on the way to Louis's: *Je suis chauve, donc je suis. I am bald, therefore I am.*

Baldosophy burdens me: Am I defined by having been born haired or by what I now don't have? Am I exhibiting my free will or am I being misled by a mysterious haired force I can't control? Will I burn in Balde's Inferno if I wear a hairpiece?

What if I like it?

Accompanied by my friend Randy Banner, who will photograph the ritual fitting of the rug, I enter Louis's. As we wait, Randy tries to take close-ups of my pate, but her autofocus lens, which has a mind of its own, refuses to focus, as if my scalp is giving off signals that say: "If you photograph me, you're stealing my soul."

When my turn comes, I enter a styling stall.

And there it sits: The Piece. Call it Zelmo. Sitting on a mannequin head. Lifeless. Formless. A wild mass of ringlets. I think I'm going to look like the tough guy in the film *Hollywood Shuffle* who begs for his hair-loosening Activator spray so his coif will remain in ringlets.

This piece is too much. It will make me look like Frank Zappa. So Louis cuts. Before he sees the mean haired streets, Zelmo needs a haircut.

He positions Zelmo on my head with double-backed tape and snips. Dampened curls tumble past my eyes for the first time in ten years; the plastic smock is littered with twice-cut hair once owned by Italian peasant women. They sold hundreds of thousands of locks of their hair so that someone could stitch them through mesh foundations and stick them on men's heads. Oh, the sacrifices of women. First they give birth, then they give hair.

Louis styles as he cuts. First he gives me a full hairline. Then some recession. I want recession.

Now, Zelmo, once damp, is drying. The ringlets turn to waves. This isn't a Frank Zappa Look. No! This is starting . . . to look . . . like . . . *ME!* when I was *EIGHTEEN!*

"Good God," I say aloud.

Is there a haired man inside my body trying to get out or is

Baldman trying to cram him back in? I can't tell. The battle for my follicular soul mounts. I sense a schizoid conversation:

"It looks great."/"It doesn't."

"It looks fantastic."/"It *can't!* I am *BALDMAN!*"

"Cut the Baldman crap!"/"Never!"

"You wish you were eighteen again."/"No I don't! No! No!"

I felt like a witness under withering cross-examination by Perry Mason.

"Isn't it true that Baldman is a sick alter ego that you created to mask your insecurities?"

"No—"

"And isn't it true that hair is what you want and now that you have it, you continue to deny it?"

"No—"

Luckily, I have Randy on my side. Or so I think. When Louis peels the piece off my head, I am au naturel again. I ask Randy what she thinks.

"I like you better bald," she says.

I am relieved. My severest female critic is on the side of right.

Louis returns with my piece, metal clips sewn into it. The clips look like miniature double-edged combs that snap together to hold the piece into fringe hair. I have four clips arrayed around the circumference of the piece. Now Louis really goes to work. With the clips anchoring it firmly, he launches into a styling and teasing frenzy without fear of the rug coming up. He cuts and teases, teases and cuts. Zelmo is slimming down and, sad to say, looking increasingly better.

As he puts the finishing touches on it, Louis gives me his commentary.

"You want a smooth, sophisticated look."

(A little like John Gotti's, Randy adds.)

"I'd get rid of the glasses, and get aviators."

"It'll last a year or two, unless you're rough with it, burn it or give it to the dog to chew."

Now Randy betrays Baldman. Seeing the final product, she says: "I like you better this way."

The Schiz Talk starts again.

"She's right, you look great."/"I see nothing."

"You *know* nothing."/"I still see a bald head."

"You *do* need glasses."/"I can't like it."

"You must. Maybe you'll score."/"Go to hell."

I tell myself, Baldman, you can't like it. You can say it looks different, but you can't like it.

TO THE WORLD

On the street, people are staring. People who aren't even looking at me are staring. *They know.* The people on the observation deck of the Empire State Building are chortling and are aiming water balloons at my head. The people on the train are hysterical. In the restaurant, I hear the waitress say, "Would you care for some dressing on your toupee?"

I glance at myself in mirrors, shocked at having a hairline. Shocked at the different shape of my head. But it feels so absolutely false. I feel as if I'm in the court of Louis XVI. I do not feel glee or triumph or studlike. It is as if a hairy UFO has landed on my head, and it's taken control of my scalp.

I go to my mother's house later that evening. It is about nine o'clock; unexpected evening doorbells scare Mom. She suspects trouble when I arrive unannounced. She opens the door, about to say, "What's wrong?" when the words stick to her tongue and she steps backward into the apartment, stunned, speechless, her hand to her heart. *Oh, God, I've given her a heart attack!* But no, she's okay.

She sits down and slowly regains the power of speech. She says it looks good and quickly rummages through her photo archives. She emerges with an album full of photos of me, taken between birth and age twenty-two. She reminisces about the hairs gone by. About the beautiful curls I sprouted at eight months. About the curls she kept short when I was ten.

"Now you look like you did when you graduated from college," she says.

She keeps looking at me in shock. Of course, she says, I look *equally* good haired and bald. Of course, it makes no difference to her whether I wear it or not.

"You always look handsome to me."

(Mothers always say that.)

I know she fears the wrath of Baldman (it wasn't until a few years ago that she first uttered the word *bald* in my presence, for fear of offending me), so she dares not say, "You look better this way."

"Day One: Baldman's Scalp Held Hostage" ends. I unsnap the clips and pull the piece off. I place Zelmo on the mannequin head and stab him with four voodoo pins to hold him in place. He sits on a chest facing my bed, staring at me as I go to sleep.

The enemy has landed and we are fighting for my very unhaired being. I fancy myself the reincarnation of Balder, the gracious Norse god murdered by the evil god Loki with a mistletoe dart.

Baldman must survive—at all costs.

OPENING MY HEAD OUT OF TOWN

The day after I bring Zelmo home, I fly to Disney World on non-scalp-related business (Baldman has to pay the rent!). The weekend is well-timed: like a Broadway show that opens out of town, I will open my false-haired head in this land of make-believe amid people who don't know me bald.

I fidget. Everywhere I go, I'm fidgeting so that the piece will look like it belongs. I carry two combs to make sure the false hair and real hair are blended well. Not a glass pane appears that I don't stop to look at for my haired reflection. The top looks full. Too full! But will Mickey care? Will Pluto pull it off? If any place is the right venue to do this, it's Disney World. If I look goofy, who'll notice?

Everyone will notice! Everyone knows! If the moorings loosen on this baby, my head will be a better attraction than Space Mountain!!!

I worry.

Do people notice anything funny when I scratch my head? Does the piece move too much?

Will Donald, Huey, Dewey and Louie steal my piece and play saloogie with it up and down Main Street?

Nyah, nyah, nyah, nyah, nyah! Baldman has a hairpiece!

By the end of the day, will Roger Rabbit be careening through Toon Town wearing my rug?

In this sterile world of pure fun, I am the pure paranoid. Disney CEO Michael Eisner will probably build something in my honor; one day, you'll be able to walk directly from Tomorrow Land to Paranoia Land.

Outside a hotel ballroom, I dance with a six-foot-tall pink hippo in a tutu. When she spins me around, her arm shifts the rug slightly. The movement feels like the continental plates shifting on my head, the sure sign of a scalpquake. Does Richter have a scale for wig movement?

I go through EPCOT Center, that land of pavilions saluting food and brotherhood and communications and space and Michael Jackson. While I careen through a simulation of the inside of the human body, I dream that Disney has built the Richard Sandomir Toupee Pavilion. Inside is a land where everyone wears fake hair, where the souvenir stands sell toupees and double-backed tape—and I'm the only one wearing my skin. Again, I'm the outsider.

"Welcome to our salute to the wonderful world of hair-pieces," I hear a soothing voice known only to me. "My, oh my, where would our world be without the toupee? Come with us on a tour of our toupee farm, where we grow false hair right out of the dry desert sand . . ."

I stand in a crowd watching Eisner (who I believe deftly covers a bald spot), George Lucas, Carrie Fisher and Mark Hamill introduce a new "Star Wars" ride. Hundreds of people look at the back of my head. They see *it*, don't they? They know I've got a toupee and they're laughing. All laughter near me is laughter at me. Mickey laughs. Minnie titters. Pluto guffaws. Even guys with toupees chuckle. I can't criticize other men's wigs. I am always tempted, as Baldman, to vigilantly comment on bad rugs, or mention that so-and-so is wearing one. But I can't for fear that the person I'm with will reply that my piece doesn't look so good, either, pal.

It comes down to this: I hate the hairpiece. It's a hairy albatross around my scalp. The fake and real hairs on the sides don't seem to want to commingle. The clips attaching the rug must be pulled tightly to anchor it, so I have a tension headache. (Excedrin Toupee Headache Number 232.) The tape holding down the front is gluey. I'm itchy half the time, paranoid all the time.

I meet a woman named Griffin Miller on this trip and we

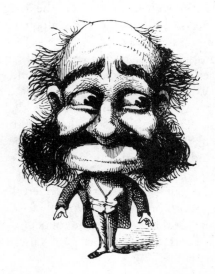

get along well. She welcomes me to a seat beside her at a press conference and we spend most of the next two days together. I wonder, as we get to know each other better, if she'll think me queer when she runs her hand through my imported Italian hair and finds metal clips that sound like cracking knuckles when they snap closed. What if we sleep together? Do I take off my clothes *and* my hair? Do I roll around the bed with the clips gnawing into my scalp so as to preserve the ruse?

When I remove it alone, late at night, I feel deep, satisfying relief when I see my shiny pate. Even with the rug on, I see a phantom vision of my scalp. When it is off, I see my natural dome. My scalp is my friend. When will I be bald?

SO, DO YOU LIKE MY HAIR?
DO YOU THINK IT'S REAL?

The questions about rugwear are many, but the basic ones are: "Does it look good/natural?" "Can I swim with it?" "Do I look younger?" and "How long will it last?"

The key question is, "What will the babes think?"

Meeting Griffin as a toupeed person, I knew I had a good test case. If she detected any funny wig business in our two days together, she didn't say. She never said a word.

A week later, we meet for a date in Brooklyn.

We chat for a few minutes before I say: "Do you like my hair?"

"Sure," she says.

"Do you like the way I style it?"

"I guess so."

"Do you think it's real?"

"It's not?"

"Nope."

"So?"

So?!?!?! What a great response. The women who count are truly of a higher species than men.

"Does it matter to you?"

"Should it?"

Wow! She's really passing the test. Either she really likes me or it truly doesn't matter to her. She could win the first Baldman Humanitarian Award.

"Honest?"

"Honest."

After dinner, I promise to take it off when we return to her apartment. During dinner, I ask, "Did you have any inkling that it wasn't my hair?"

"A little," she says, "but I wasn't sure."

"Did anything give it away?"

"No, but my ex-husband wore one and it was the worst toupee ever. And he spent good money—my money—on it. But each one he got was worse than the one before. It was long and stringy and I couldn't believe he thought it looked good."

"So in comparison . . ."

"Yours looks great. And you really can't tell unless someone tells you it's a piece."

"Really?"

"Really."

I can't believe this woman! She's too good to be true. I might as well marry her right here!

Back in her apartment, I hurry to the bathroom with my comb and pick. I unsnap the clips, peel off the tape and put Zelmo aside. I tease and comb my real hair, which gets tangled and unmanageable under the piece.

I put the piece on a table. Later, I will move it to my coat pocket; I don't want her hairnivorous and evil cat to chew it up, much as Tramp the dog did to William Frawley's rug in *My Three Sons*.

I walk slowly into the living room.

The unveiling is seconds away.

This *could* doom the relationship.

Her reaction will make the difference between getting thrown out of the apartment and, well, you know . . .

She is seated on her couch.

I've never done this before.

My shaking is barely perceptible.

She looks up and smiles beatifically at my bald head. I feel like Robert Redford when Glenn Close, in white, stands and looks on as he slugs a homer in *The Natural.*

"Ah," she said. "Now *that's* better."

Perfection.

IT COST YOU $850? I THOUGHT YOU SAID $8.50

And now, "Three Haired Men and a Baldie."

(The scene opens with Baldman meeting Dave outside a Manhattan Chinese restaurant.)

Dave (almost dropping his newspaper): My philosophy is if you want to buy a piece, at least get a good one.

Baldman (defensively): So you don't like it?

Dave: What did you spend for it?

Baldman: Eight-fifty.

Dave: Is that a cheap one?

Baldman: No, the prices range from about five to twelve.

Dave: And for eight fifty you get a good one?

Baldman: Right.

Dave: Hmmmm.

(A Volvo, with Arthur and David in it, glides past. Arthur is laughing hysterically and pointing. He is so distracted that he pulls into the exit ramp of a garage. All four enter the restaurant. Arthur, Dave and David are laughing.)

Baldman (embarrassed that his friends are being so raucous, says to the maitre d'): Do you have a table in a darker area?

Maitre d': No. No table for four. Only six.

Baldman: We'll eat like six.

Maitre d': No. No. Sit there.

(He leads the foursome to a brightly lit table next to two

beautiful women. All four sit and speak loudly enough for all surrounding tables to hear.)

Arthur: That's the worst rug I've ever seen! Really terrible!

Baldman: Oh, come on.

David (staring intently at Baldman's hairline. He shakes his head from side to side in disbelief): It just doesn't look like your hair is growing out of your head.

Baldman: You really think it's bad, huh? You wouldn't say that if you didn't know me.

Arthur: If I saw you for the first time, I'd say, "That guy is wearing a bad toupee."

David: Yep.

Dave: Uh-huh.

Arthur: Tell me you're not going to go out and pick up women with that on, are you?

Baldman: I did that already.

Arthur: And she went out with you despite the fact that you looked like a ridiculous asshole?

Baldman: Yup.

David: Was she blind?

Baldman: No, either she didn't notice or she didn't care. That's why women are a higher species than you goons.

(The food comes and conversation veers to idle chatter, before it returns to the rug on Baldman's head.)

Dave: How does it attach?

Baldman: With clips that snap into place like this. Listen closely.

(The four lean in to listen to the snaps that sound like knuckles cracking. The three cringe and moan audibly.)

David: Oh, Jesus!

Dave: And how does it attach up front?

Baldman: With tape.

(Baldman raises up front to show the taped section.)

David: No, no, don't do that!

Baldman (giving the *Honeymooners* Raccoon salute with the piece): Woo-woo!

Dave: Now how much did you pay for that again?

Baldman: Eight hundred fifty dollars.

Dave (pondering his pricing misperception): I thought you said eight dollars and fifty cents! I thought you got it from a novelty store. I was thinking that you shouldn't have spent any more than ten bucks on it. Twelve at the most.

Baldman: Well, you're an extremely stupid person, aren't you?

Dave: Why didn't you get one that's fuller, that has no recession?

Baldman: Well, it would be a shock to everyone. I should have some recession. I'm thirty-two. If I had a big, full head of hair it wouldn't look natural.

Arthur (laughing): Oh, right, it wouldn't look natural. We wouldn't have thought of that!

(Baldman exits for a few minutes to adjust the piece in the men's room to bring the hairline forward.)

Dave: That looks better, but the front only looks slightly more natural than before, which doesn't say much.

David: It still doesn't look as if it's growing out of your head.

Arthur: It's still an incredibly lousy piece.

Baldman: Now, really, guys, I don't think you're being objective. You know me and it's a shock to see me with hair. Baldman was born in the office we all worked in, so you can't make a good decision on this. If you didn't know me, would you be so critical?

Arthur: Of course we would.

David: Yup.

Dave: Uh-huh.

David (staring intently at the piece again): I like you better bald.

Baldman: Thanks, that's the nicest thing I've heard you say yet.

(The four leave the restaurant and talk for several minutes outside.)

David (continuing to stare at the piece): It looks worse in the sunlight.

Baldman: Okay, I'm going. You can say some even nastier things about me when I'm gone.

Arthur: No, we pretty much said everything to your face—and your fake hair.

EPILOGUE: BALDMAN TRIUMPHANT

I've had enough of Zelmo. After a few weeks, I've had it. I'll admit people didn't stop in their tracks to stare in amazement at the folly of my false follicles, or twist their heads 360 degrees to make sure they didn't miss my head the first time, but it is enough that I sense the folly. If wearing this does nothing for me, it's worthless. If I keep seeing and wishing for a bald head despite the presence of my Italian hair donor's snipped-off curls, I don't need it.

Every minute Zelmo is clamped onto me, I feel I'm committing a crime against myself: felonious (and silly) impersonation of a person with hair. I act differently with it. I walk differently with it. I even bought a brush, my first in fifteen or twenty years, and new combs. When I furtively leave my apartment, I hope no one is walking the halls or outside the building; I pray my neighbors will not bear witness to what George Bush might call "the rug thing."

I am ashamed of me with hair because for me, being haired is an unnatural state. I'm not the person I really am when I cross the line to join the hairists. I crave my natural pate every minute it smothers, sweats and cries beneath the rug.

Zelmo never had a chance. Even if he had made a dramatic change in my life, he was going to lose. The bald gods were allied against him from the start.

He came into this world as dead hair on a field of mesh.

He shall leave as vanquished protein.

INDEX